NOV 3 ~ 2005

NEENAH PUB
NEENAH, W

WITHDRAWN

D0946986

SOMERSIZE
APPETIZERS

Also by SUZANNE SOMERS

Touch Me

Keeping Secrets

Wednesday's Children

Suzanne Somers' Eat Great, Lose Weight

Suzanne Somers' Get Skinny on Fabulous Food

After the Fall

365 Ways to Change Your Life

Suzanne Somers' Eat, Cheat, and Melt the Fat Away

Somersize Desserts

Suzanne Somers' Fast and Easy

The Sexy Years

Somersize Chocolate

Suzanne Somers' Slim and Sexy Forever

Somersize Cocktails

SOMERSIZE
APPETIZERS
SUZANNE SOMERS

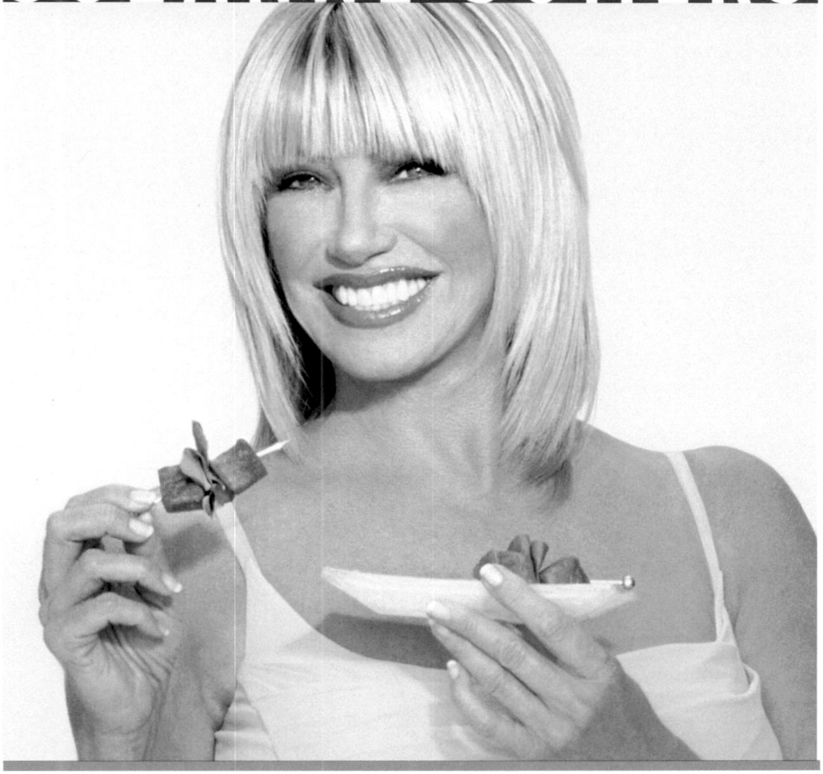

30

Scintillating

Starters to

Tantalize

Your

Tastebuds

at Every

Occasion

CROWN PUBLISHERS, NEW YORK

Copyright © 2005 by Suzanne Somers
Photographs copyright 2005 © by Jeff Katz

All rights reserved.
Published in the United States by Crown Publishers, New York, an imprint of the
Crown Publishing Group, a division of Random House, Inc., New York.
www.crownpublishig.com

CROWN is a trademark and the Crown colophon is a registered trademark of Random House, Inc.

Library of Congress Cataloging-in-Publication Data
Somers, Suzanne
    Somersize appetizers : 30 scintillating starters to tantalize your tastebuds at every occasion /
Suzanne Somers.
    Includes index.
    1. Appetizers.   2. Low-carbohydrate diet—Recipes.   I. Title.
TX740.S6235   2005
641.8'74—dc22   2005015380

ISBN-13: 978-1-4000-5331-5
ISBN-10: 1-4000-5331-5

Printed in the United States of America

Design by Lauren Dong

10   9   8   7   6   5   4   3   2   1

First Edition

641.812
50545

This book is for Al Lowman, my literary agent. You breathed life into every day.

Your fight for each breath inspired me and taught me to regard each day as a blessing.

I send you my breath and my energy as a small token of my appreciation for all the love

and support you have given me all these years. I love you and will always miss you.

5

Contents

Acknowledgments

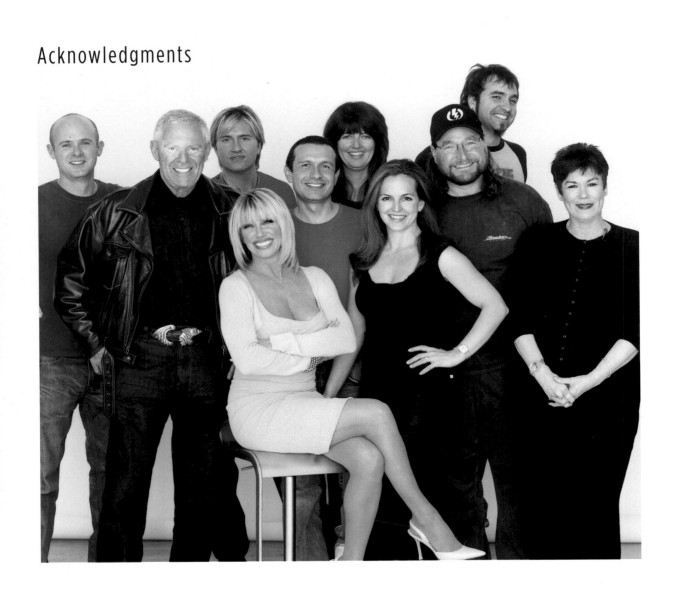

As with all my Somersize books, Caroline Somers has been right by my side. Whether we are testing recipes in the kitchen, making sure the text reads just right, designing a new look for the photos, or selecting just the right platter, you are my Somersize ace. I am so lucky to have you in my life in business and as my daughter-in-law. I love you dearly.

To Louise Charbonneau, it was a pleasure to spend so many days with you in the kitchen surrounded by incredible food. Your creativity and innovative ideas for taste combinations have enriched my cooking and I thank you for your excellence. Thank you to your assistants, Jewels Elmore, Jennifer Fox, and Milena Robertson, for all their prepping to make the photographs so special.

To my favorite photographer and dear friend, Jeff Katz, thank you for stretching outside of the box and making this new look work. You nailed it. I love the food photography, and your gorgeous lighting on the cover shot makes me feel twenty years younger! Thanks to your team and my buddies, Jack Coyier, Victor Boghossian, Andy Strauss, and Stuart Gow.

To Denise Vivaldo and Cindie Flannigan of Food Fanatics, my food stylists extraordinaire, you made the food look like art. It's picture perfect and I love the humor you bring to a set.

To my prop stylist, Laurie Baer, and her team of Claire Harbo and Katie Hofsomer, thank you for your sense of simplicity in making this look artistic and still a reflection of me.

To my Secretary of Hair—Mooney, if I could only be as gorgeous as you are! At least I have you to get my hair just right at any hour of the day or night.

To Barbara Farman on makeup, I am so pleased with the fresh and clean look you helped me to achieve. You are a pro.

To Xavier Cabrera on wardrobe, you have me pressed, pulled, and tugged in all the right places.

To Marsha Yanchuck, for being my watchdog all these years, and for great proofreading. To Julie Turkel, thanks for keeping me scheduled to the minute. And to my assistant, Liz Kozakowski, you are my Speedy Gonzalez and you keep me sane.

To Kristin Kiser, who has been my editor for too many books to count, congratulations on your beautiful baby girl. And to Lindsey Moore, who stepped in as editor in Kristin's absence, you made the transition seamless and you're a pleasure to work with. Thank you for doing such a great job.

To my champions at Crown—Jenny Frost, Steve Ross, Philip Patrick, Tina Constable, and Tammy Blake, there is no one with whom I would rather work.

And thank you to the production team at Crown—Amy Boorstein, Trisha Howell, Leta Evanthes, and Lauren Dong. To Dan Rembert, who did the cover design, we went round and round on this, and I think you landed in just the right spot.

Thank you to my attorney, Marc Chamlin, for ushering through all the legal affairs with finesse and diplomacy.

Thank you to Al Lowman, my literary agent, for believing in me and for being a huge light force in my life. I love you and think of you in heaven, smiling and laughing with your goofy laugh. God bless you.

And to my husband, Alan Hamel, because none of this would be, nor would it be any fun, without you!

My sincere thanks to all of you. There is one woman on the cover, but you all make it happen.

Introduction

Appetizers are the sexy little bites that tantalize your taste buds before the meal. An appetizer can be a passed hors d'oeuvre, like finger food, or a sit-down first course in a smaller portion than is customary for an entrée. Either way, this first section is aptly named, since the appetizer is the introduction to the meal. It sets the mood with its taste and presentation. It whets the appetite, without killing it (if done right), and leaves your guests anticipating what is to come.

My favorite part of any party that I host or attend is the cocktail hour. Not because I'm a lush—but because I love the freedom to mill about with all the guests, and to enjoy savory little passed bites that float from the kitchen. The tone for the evening is set in this hour. Whether serving something as simple as a margarita and a bowl of chips with salsa or as fancy as the finest champagne and caviar on roasted fingerling potatoes, a good hostess knows how to cue the evening with the presentation of the appetizers and drinks. I've written a book called *Somersize Cocktails,* which has fun and delicious drink recipes—the perfect partners to the appetizers in this book—that make for a memorable cocktail hour.

In this book, I have focused mostly on passed appetizers, although many of these dishes can be served as a sit-down first course. When I serve appetizers, I like small bites. Some appetizers that are too large can disintegrate with the first bite and spill on your clothing. It's also awkward when you're talking with guests to have large bites of food in your mouth. So I love a perfect little bite, like my Clams Gratin with Pancetta and Arugula or Artichoke Leaves with Tarragon Aïoli and Shaved Parmesan. Others, favorites such as Sweet Shrimp with Hot Green Chutney and Wild Mushroom Risotto in Mushroom Caps, are wonderful as two to three bites.

Here's how I know if I've done my job right as a hostess. When I serve an appetizer to my guests, I watch the eyes. When they see the tray, there should be a small lift in the eyebrow that says, "Hmmm, that looks interesting." This lets me know my presentation is right on. Then I watch the eyes again as that sumptuous bite enters his or her mouth. If the eyes widen and I hear a gasp, followed by a scrunched face that screams, "Oh, that is so good," that's when I know I've hit my mark.

Appetizers should be exciting. Even when I dine

in a restaurant, I sometimes order completely off the appetizer menu. The tastes are so intriguing, and I love sampling so many flavors from the kitchen without committing to an entire entrée. Now several restaurants are adopting this style of small plates so that you can experience many tastes.

What are the elements that make a good appetizer? Presentation is essential. The level of formality of your meal will dictate the types of serving trays or platters for your appetizers. For a poolside party, Chili-Braised Pork with Tomatillo Salsa would look fabulous served on a brightly colored tray set out alongside tall glasses of Ginger Lime Cooler. This says casual and fun. For an evening event, you might choose to pass these spicy colorful morsels on a plain silver tray with a Lychee Martini to make the evening more upscale, but the flavors let your guests know the food is anything but ordinary.

When the food is perfectly prepared, the appetizer itself is the art. As you can see from the photos in this book, arranging the food in sleek patterns makes for a stunning presentation. These designs on a plain tray are an elegant way to set a mood. Trays may also be adorned with a small flower or nosegay, or with a simple herb or fruit garnish. This is where you get to express yourself as a host or hostess. Look for edible, organic flowers at the farmers' market, or grow some herbs in a pot by the kitchen window. Tie them off with a string of raffia for a rustic look or a thin satin ribbon for something more romantic. Use a fancy food cutter to make interesting shapes

with vegetables. Let your creativity show. This is your chance to shine.

When it comes to the food preparation for your appetizers, get as much done as you can in advance. Clean and chop earlier in the day, or the night before. Make the cold dipping sauces in advance; they will keep until your event begins. Chop your meat, poultry, or fish, but save the actual cooking or assembling until right before your guests arrive to keep things as fresh as possible. When appetizers are assembled too early they can become oxidized and turn color. This is not appetizing and is a waste of all your hard work! For instance, with my divine Rock Shrimp Salad on Cucumber Rounds, prepare the cucumber the morning of by scoring it and slicing it into rounds. Wrap the pieces in a moist paper towel and store inside a plastic bag. Prepare the rock shrimp salad next and keep it in the refrigerator in a sealed container. Then, chop all the garnishes and set them aside. Assemble as close as possible to your guests' arrival. The assembly is quick since everything is all ready for you. This gives you a chance to give the rock shrimp salad another good stir before you place perfect dollops onto the precut cucumber rounds. On the other hand, if you were to place the shrimp salad onto the cucumber rounds and then set the whole tray in the fridge for two hours, the appetizers would not look as fresh and appealing when it's time to serve. Timing is by far the most challenging part of entertaining, and the only way to perfect it is with practice.

The appetizers you will find in this book range

from the very simple, like Parmesan Crisps with Prosciutto and Arugula, to the more time consuming, like Lobster Thermidor with a homemade glaçage. Either way, each step is carefully laid out to help you succeed every time. Exotic ingredients may be replaced with more readily available ones, and I have given options for doing so in each recipe.

Somersize is synonymous with healthy living by eliminating refined sugars and using real ingredients, such as protein, healthy fats, fresh vegetables, fruits, and whole grains. The result is wholesome, delicious food that tastes incredible. These recipes follow the Somersize guidelines. For my many Somersize loyalists, you know that Level One means the food can be eaten during the weight-loss phase of the program. Almost Level One means the item is just slightly outside the guidelines for weight loss, and can be enjoyed once you are steadily losing. Level Two foods are for maintenance, when you have lost all the weight you want and will continue to keep your trim figure for years to come. In place of sugar, I use my signature sweetener, SomerSweet. It's available at SuzanneSomers.com. You may also substitute sugar or any sweetener you like.

So many appetizers revolve around a cracker, a toast point, a slice of bread, or a chip as the base. I have tried to come up with many alternatives to the white flour carbohydrate base of the hors d'oeuvre.

In this book, you'll find innovative ways to use mushroom caps, artichoke hearts, Parmesan crisps, lettuce cups, skewers, and many more finger foods that can be picked up and eaten cleanly and neatly. Plus, you'll find more offbeat suggestions, such as passing a tray of demitasse cups filled with Lobster Bisque Cappuccino. They look just like frothy cappuccinos, but what a treat to have a small taste of rich and delicious soup. Now that's a catapult from the basic cheese and cracker!

Most of these recipes are written with eight guests in mind. I usually figure two appetizers per person, so many of the recipes yield sixteen pieces. Adjust to your style of entertaining. You may want to make several different appetizers or stick with only one in order to keep your to-do list easier. You are the orchestra leader of your party and you get to make the decisions.

Somersizer or not, these appetizers will entice your most discerning guests. They are unique and exciting, delicious and fresh. Wait until you stun your guests with spoonfuls of Spicy Tomato Sorbet with Cracked Black Pepper and Basil. It's a wow! Have fun with these amazing creations and make sure to pair them with your favorite drinks from my companion book, *Somersize Cocktails*. Have fun, and enjoy the party!

SUZANNE SOMERS

SOMERSIZE
APPETIZERS

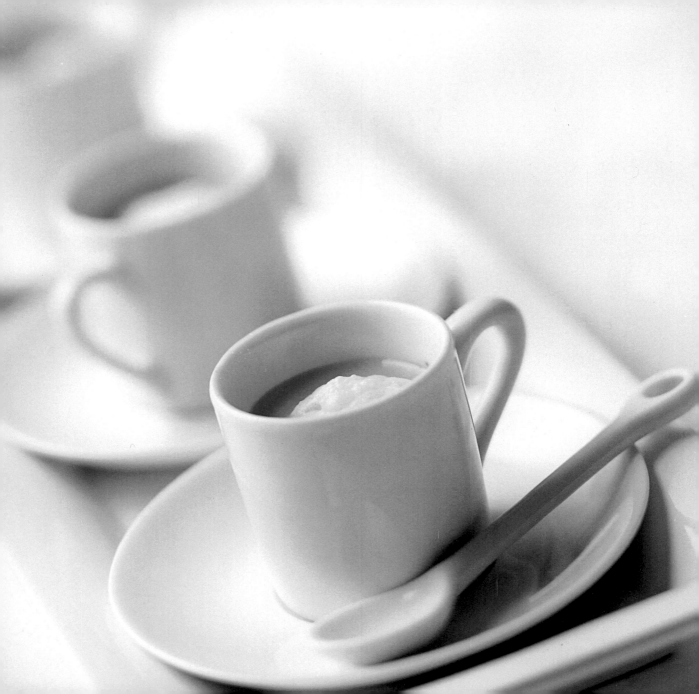

LOBSTER BISQUE CAPPUCCINO

SERVES 8

Caroline and Bruce had a birthday party for me and this was one of the fabulous appetizers. It looks like a cappuccino in a demitasse cup with a foamy, frothy top, but when you have a sip, your mouth gets an out-of-this-world surprise of lobster bisque. Rich, creamy, and delicious. For a passed hors d'oeuvre I serve this without the lobster chunks so it can be sipped without a spoon. As a sit-down course I add the chunks.

Remove the lobster meat from the tails and claws and set aside. Reserve the lobster shells.

Heat a large stockpot on medium. Add 1 tablespoon of the butter, the onion, celery, and bell pepper. Cook for about 10 minutes to let the vegetables slowly sweat. Add the lobster shells to the pot, mashing with a wooden spoon to break up the shells and release the flavor. Add the tomato paste, stirring with the shells until it begins to caramelize.

Add the white wine to deglaze the pan. Bring to a boil, then lower the heat to a simmer and let reduce by half. Add the chicken broth and let cook over medium heat until it boils. Then lower the heat to a simmer for 10 minutes. Add the cream and reduce the entire soup again by half.

Strain through a medium sieve, pressing the shells and vegetables to extract all the flavor. Pour the strained bisque into a clean pot and bring back to a simmer. Adjust the seasoning with salt and pepper. Using a whisk, incorporate the remaining 3 tablespoons of butter into the soup.

Using a milk frother, foam the milk until light and fluffy. (If you do not have a milk frother, whip a small amount of heavy cream to soft peaks instead.) To serve as a tray-passed appetizer, fill demitasse cups two-thirds full and top with a dollop of foamed milk. Serve immediately. To serve as a first course at a sit-down dinner, cut up the lobster meat into small chunks and fill each cup with a few chunks of lobster meat. Add bisque until the cup is two-thirds full and top with a dollop of foamed milk. Serve immediately.

---

1 whole lobster, 1^1/$_2$–2 pounds, cooked and cleaned (with the shell)

4 tablespoons (^{1}/$_2$ stick) butter

1 onion, sliced

1 stalk celery, sliced

1 red bell pepper, seeded and sliced

2 tablespoons tomato paste

2 cups white wine

4 cups chicken broth

2 cups heavy cream

Sea salt and freshly ground black pepper

1 cup nonfat milk (or heavy cream for Level One)

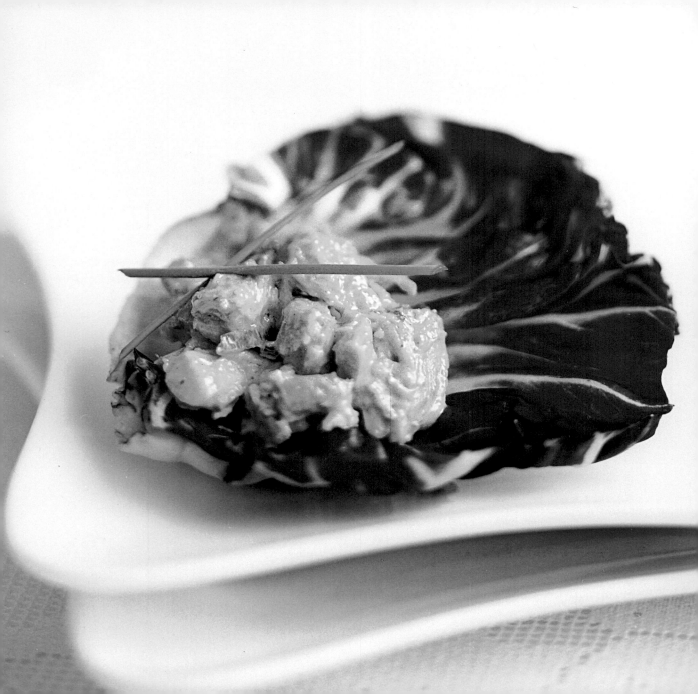

RADICCHIO CUPS WITH CURRIED CHICKEN

MAKES 16 CUPS

Chicken salad sounds so simple, but this flavor is anything but. The exotic taste of red curry paste gives it a kick. It is beautifully served in radicchio cups.

To make the marinade, in a sealable plastic bag, mix the curry paste and curry powder with 2 tablespoons of the olive oil and the juice from ½ of the lime. Place the chicken into the marinade and refrigerate for 30 minutes, turning once to evenly coat.

Preheat the oven to 375 degrees.

Place an ovenproof sauté pan over medium heat and add the remaining tablespoon of olive oil. Sear the chicken for 3 minutes on each side. Add the chicken broth and bring to a boil. Cover the pan with a lid and place into the oven until the chicken is cooked through, about 30 minutes. Remove the chicken from the pan and allow to cool, reserving the juices. When cool enough to handle, chop the chicken into small pieces and reserve 1 tablespoon of the liquid.

In a small bowl, mix together the mayonnaise and the reserved liquid. Add the chicken and season to taste with salt, pepper, and a squeeze of lime juice.

Use each raddicchio leaf as a cup. Trim with kitchen scissors, if necessary. Spoon the chicken filling into radicchio cups, garnish with a crisscross of chives, and serve immediately.

2 tablespoons Thai red curry paste

1 teaspoon dried yellow curry powder

3 tablespoons extra-virgin olive oil

1 lime

3 chicken thighs, boned

1 cup chicken broth

¼ cup mayonnaise

Sea salt and freshly ground black pepper

3 heads radicchio, leaves washed and separated

Chives, for garnish

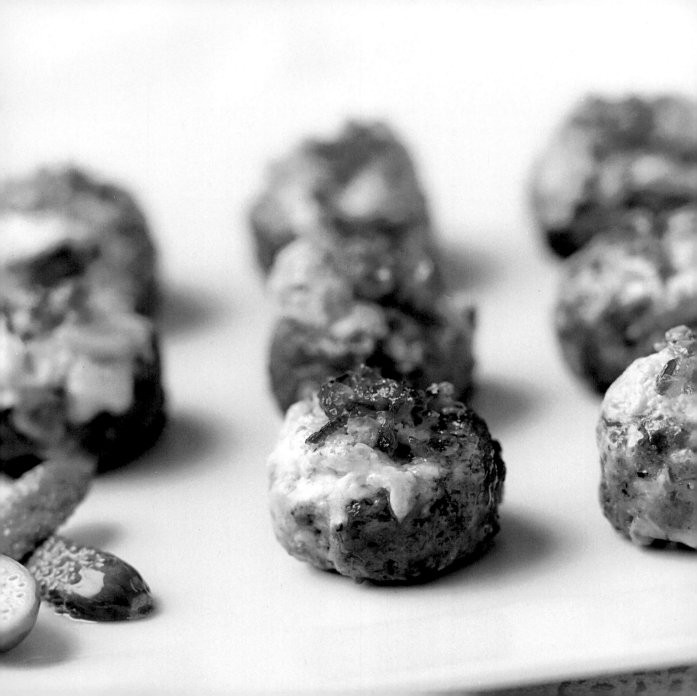

MINI BURGERS WITH GORGONZOLA and CARAMELIZED ONIONS

MAKES 16

What could be better than a burger with Gorgonzola and onions? Now it's bite-size as a special appetizer treat.

1 pound ground beef
1/4 cup finely minced onion (preferably Vidalia or Maui)
1 egg
Sea salt and freshly ground black pepper
1 tablespoon extra-virgin olive oil
6 ounces Gorgonzola, cut into 12 thin slices
1 recipe Caramelized Onions (recipe follows)

In a mixing bowl, combine the beef, minced onion, egg, salt, and pepper. Form into 1-inch balls, then flatten slightly to form patties and set aside.

In a sauté pan over medium-high heat, add the olive oil and sear the burgers until they are crispy and brown, about 2 minutes per side. Remove from the heat and transfer to a baking sheet.

Preheat the broiler. Top the burgers with Gorgonzola and place under the broiler to melt the cheese. Top with caramelized onions and serve immediately.

CARAMELIZED ONIONS

Extra-virgin olive oil
1 onion, preferably Maui, very thinly sliced

In a medium sauté pan over medium-high heat, add olive oil to coat the pan. Add the onion slices in one layer and cook until they become brown and golden, 7 to 10 minutes. Once they begin to caramelize on the bottom, stir and turn to caramelize the tops. Lower the heat and continue to cook until soft and caramelized throughout.

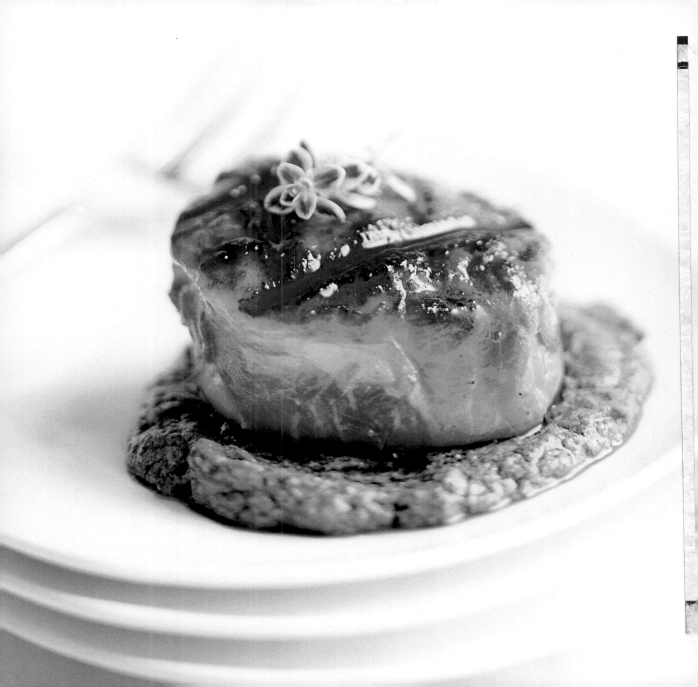

GRILLED SCALLOPS WRAPPED IN PROSCIUTTO WITH BASIL-PARSLEY PISTOU

MAKES 16

I love the combination of tender scallops with crisp prosciutto. Not only are they delicious, but they are also quick to throw together and grill. If using the very large sea scallops, quarter them to make into nice bite size pieces. Smaller scallops can be used whole. You may also use prawns for this recipe instead of scallops. The Basil-Parsely Pistou is just the right topper. Serve this on salad greens and you'll have a lovely entrée salad.

Preheat grill to high.

Loosely wrap each scallop with ½ piece prosciutto. Season with salt and pepper, drizzle with olive oil, and secure on a skewer.

Grill the wrapped scallops until evenly browned, about 2 to 3 minutes on each side. Remove from the grill and serve on a small puddle of Basil–Parsley Pistou.

4 large sea scallops, quartered, or 16 whole scallops
8 thin slices prosciutto
Sea salt and freshly ground black pepper
Extra-virgin olive oil
16 wooden skewers soaked in water
1 recipe Basil–Parsley Pistou (recipe follows

BASIL-PARSLEY PISTOU

MAKES ABOUT 1 CUP

Set aside a small bowl filled with ice and water. Bring a small pot of water to a boil and add the basil leaves for 30 seconds to soften. Remove immediately and plunge the leaves into the ice water. After 30 to 60 seconds, remove the leaves from the ice bath, squeeze out excess water, and place into a blender. Add the remaining ingredients and purée until smooth.

2 cups basil leaves, loosely packed
½ cup flat-leaf parsley, loosely packed
½ cup freshly grated Parmesan cheese
¼ cup toasted pine nuts (omit for Level One)
¾ cup extra-virgin olive oil
1 clove garlic, minced
½ teaspoon sea salt
Freshly ground black pepper

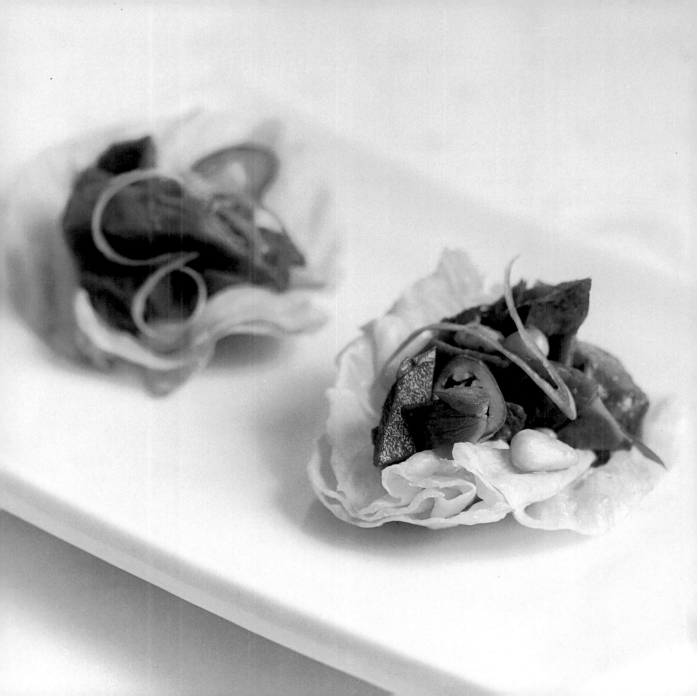

MINI LETTUCE CUPS WITH MINCED DUCK

MAKES 16 CUPS

When you serve duck at a party, your guests feel very special. What they don't know is that cooking these duck legs is as easy as preparing chicken legs. This appetizer is incredible: rich duck in cold, crispy lettuce with a crunch of pine nuts. Yum!

Preheat the oven to 375 degrees.

Season the duck liberally with salt and pepper, then coat the duck in 1 tablespoon of the oil. Place the duck into a roasting pan skin side down. Place into the oven and roast for 30 minutes, then turn the duck and roast for another 30 minutes. When fully cooked, remove from the pan and set aside to cool.

Prepare 16 lettuce cups by cutting leaves into 3 to 4-inch round disks using kitchen scissors. Set aside.

In a sauté pan over medium heat, add the remaining tablespoon of the olive oil and the garlic. Toast the garlic until lightly browned. Set aside.

Mince the duck, including the skin, into small pieces and place into a bowl. Add the toasted garlic and remaining ingredients and toss until combined. Adjust the seasoning. Spoon into lettuce rounds and serve immediately.

4 duck legs

Sea salt and freshly ground black pepper

2 tablespoons extra-virgin olive oil

1 head iceberg lettuce, washed

1 clove garlic, minced

2 scallions, chopped

1 tablespoon soy sauce

1 teaspoon sesame oil

1/4 teaspoon chili paste

Juice from 1/2 lime

2 tablespoons toasted pine nuts
(omit for Level One)

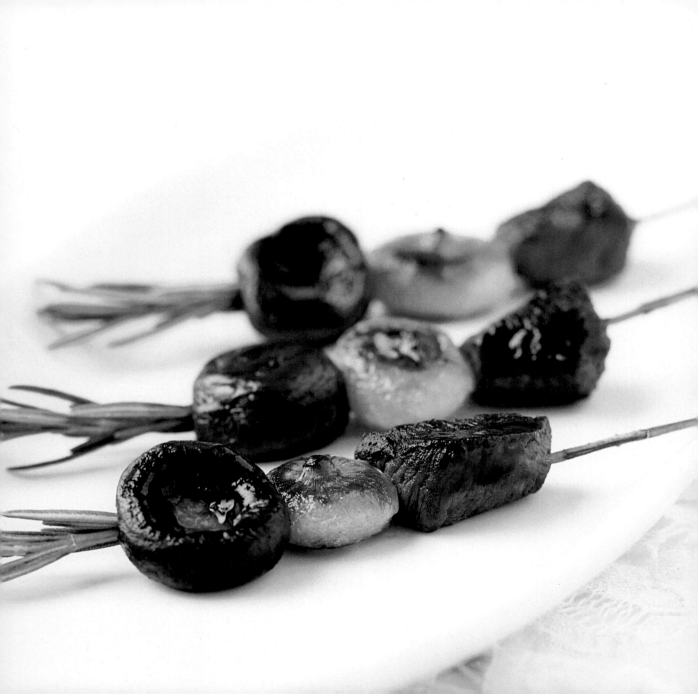

BEEF BOURGUIGNONNE BROCHETTES

MAKES 16 SKEWERS

Beef bourguignonne is the French version of pot roast. It's the ultimate comfort food. In this recipe, the tasty bites of meat are placed onto skewers with mushrooms and caramelized onions for a rich and decadent appetizer. Veal demi-glace is a rich stock that works wonders in your sauces. It's available at gourmet markets. For a beautiful presentation, use fresh rosemary stems as skewers.

Season the meat with salt and pepper. In a large sauté pan over medium-high heat, add 1 tablespoon of olive oil and the beef. Sear on each side until brown, about 2 minutes per side. Remove the pan from the heat. Transfer the meat to a bowl and set aside. Reserve the pan to make a sauce with the tasty bits on the bottom.

Place the pan back onto medium heat. Heat another tablespoon of oil, then add the onions and whole mushrooms. Cook, stirring occasionally, until the onions are golden, 10 to 12 minutes. Deglaze the pan by adding the red wine. Scrape bits from the bottom of the pan with a wooden spoon to release the flavor. Reduce the wine by half. Add the veal demi-glace and reduce again by half. Return the meat to the pan and add the butter. Adjust the seasonings to taste. Place 1 piece of beef, 1 onion, and 1 mushroom on each skewer and ladle a little sauce over the top. Serve immediately.

$1/2$ pound beef tenderloin
Sea salt and freshly ground
black pepper
Extra-virgin olive oil
16 cipolline onions
(button size, peeled
and cleaned whole)
16 cremini mushrooms
(or regular white
mushrooms)
$1/2$ cup red wine
$1/2$ cup veal demi-glace
(or beef broth)
1 tablespoon butter
16 wooden skewers (or fresh
rosemary stems)

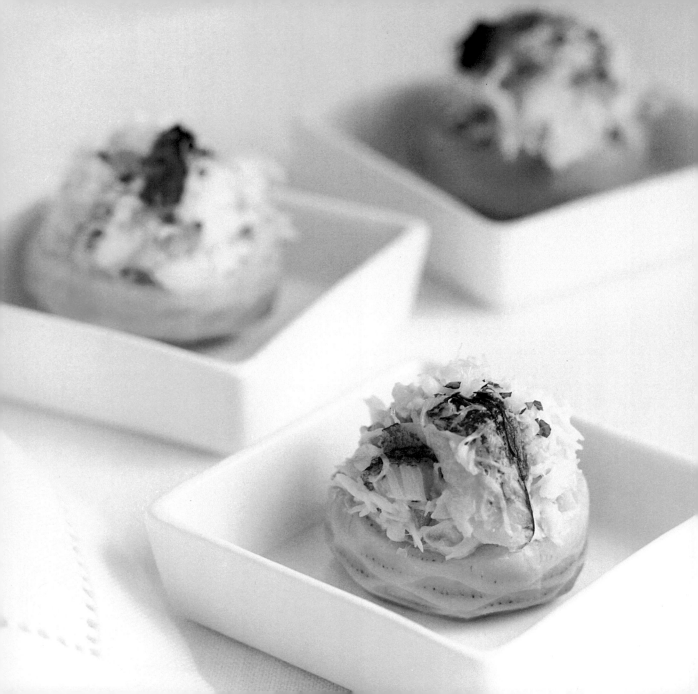

ARTICHOKE BOTTOMS WITH DUNGENESS CRAB SALAD

SERVES 8

Artichokes are one of my favorite foods. So is crab. Now the two are together in this divine combination. Artichokes have genders: the males are pointy and the females are round. I prefer the females because they have a better flavor. You may also use canned artichoke bottoms. Whether using freshly steamed or canned, serve a whole artichoke bottom topped with crab for a sit-down first course. For a passed hors d'oeuvre, simply slice the artichoke bottom into triangular pieces and top with the crab salad.

Pick through the crabmeat to make sure there are no shells. Place into a mixing bowl and add all the ingredients except the artichokes and parsley. Stir to combine and season with salt and pepper. Fill each artichoke bottom with crab mixture. Garnish with chopped parsley and serve immediately.

$1/2$ pound fresh Dungeness crabmeat
$1/4$ cup finely diced celery
$1/4$ cup finely diced onion
Sea salt and freshly ground black pepper
Juice from $1/2$ lemon
$1/4$ cup mayonnaise
16 artichoke bottoms canned in water, or 8 freshly steamed
Chopped flat-leaf parsley, for garnish

27

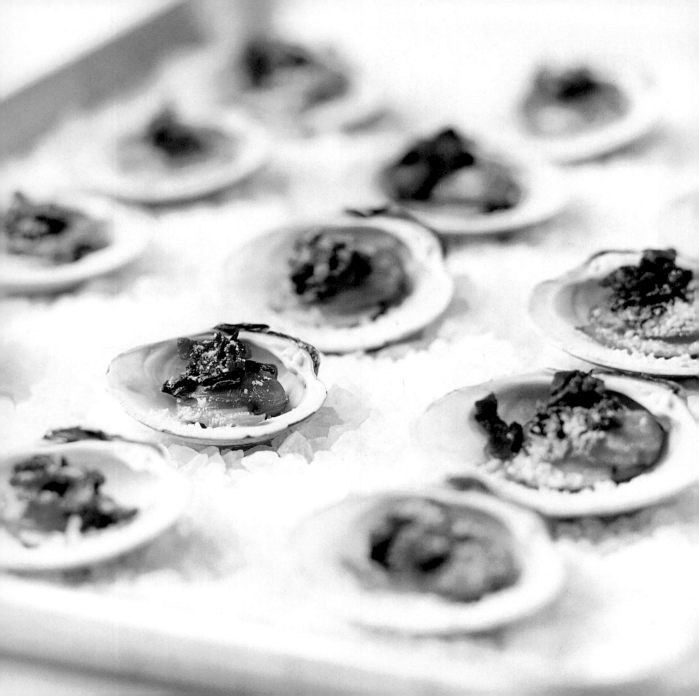

CLAMS GRATIN WITH PANCETTA and ARUGULA

MAKES 16

Wonderful, sweet, oceany bites of clams balanced with salty pancetta, spicy arugula, and a wisp of Parmesan. The perfect little bite.

Preheat the boiler.

In a large sauté pan over medium-high heat, warm enough olive oil to coat the pan. Add the garlic and allow it to brown. Add the clams and toss in the oil to coat. Deglaze with the wine. Season with salt and pepper. Cover the pan and cook until the clams open. When they are opened, remove them from the heat immediately and allow to cool. (Discard any clams that do not open.) When the clams are cool enough to handle, discard the top half of the shell. Reserve the clam broth. Place the clams in their shells onto a baking sheet.

Wilt the arugula in a hot sauté pan with a bit of olive oil. Remove from the heat to cool. Finely chop the arugula.

Spoon a little of the clam broth over the top of the clams and sprinkle with the pancetta, arugula, and Parmesan cheese. Place under the broiler for 3 minutes. Serve immediately.

Extra-virgin olive oil
1 clove garlic, smashed
16 to 18 cherrystone clams, or whatever is available fresh
1/2 cup white wine
Sea salt and freshly ground black pepper
1 cup arugula
1/4 cup pancetta (or bacon), cooked and rendered until crispy, crumbled
Freshly grated Parmesan cheese, for garnish

29

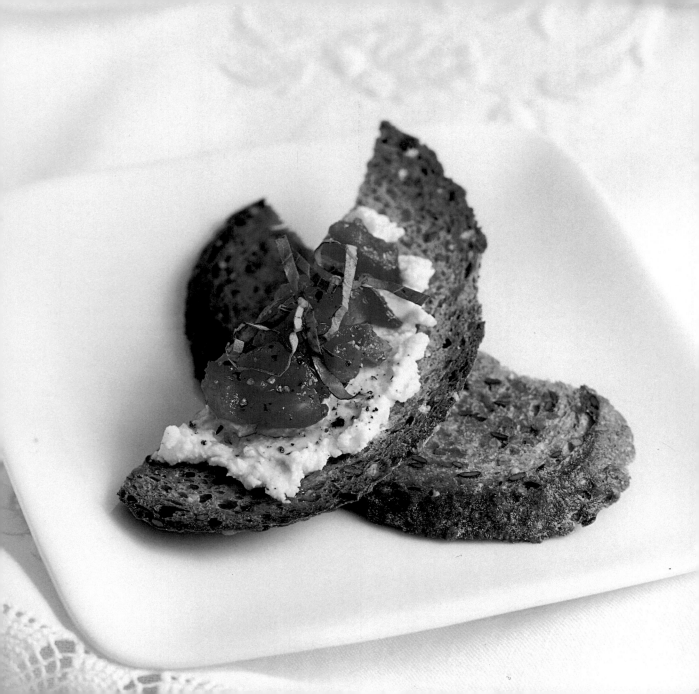

WHOLE-WHEAT CROSTINI WITH GOAT CHEESE and CANDIED TOMATO RELISH

LEVEL TWO

MAKES 16

A perfect piece of crusty whole-grain bread with a high-quality goat cheese is nothing short of perfection. In this recipe I add a candied tomato relish as the topper.

Chop the candied tomatoes into small pieces. Mix in a bowl with the basil and olive oil and season with salt and pepper.

Thinly slice the bread to create 2 x 4-inch pieces. Brush the bread with olive oil and toast in the oven or a toaster oven until lightly browned. Smear with the goat cheese and top with the tomato relish.

6 Candied Roma Tomatoes
   (recipe follows)
2 tablespoons julienned basil
Extra-virgin olive oil
Sea salt and freshly ground
   black pepper
1 loaf crusty whole-grain
   bread
6 ounces fresh goat cheese

CANDIED ROMA TOMATOES

PRO/FATS AND
VEGGIES—LEVEL ONE

MAKES 12

A Somersize staple; this method makes any lousy tomato taste great.

Preheat oven to 350 degrees.

Halve the tomatoes lengthwise and squeeze out most of the seeds. Coat in olive oil, sprinkle with SomerSweet, and season liberally with salt. Place tomatoes cut side down on a baking sheet or roasting pan. Roast for about 1 hour, or until the skin becomes crinkly and slightly browned. Remove from the oven and peel off the skin (optional). Serve warm or store in an airtight container until ready to use.

6 Roma tomatoes
1/4 cup olive oil
1/4 teaspoon SomerSweet
   (or 1 teaspoon sugar)
Sea salt

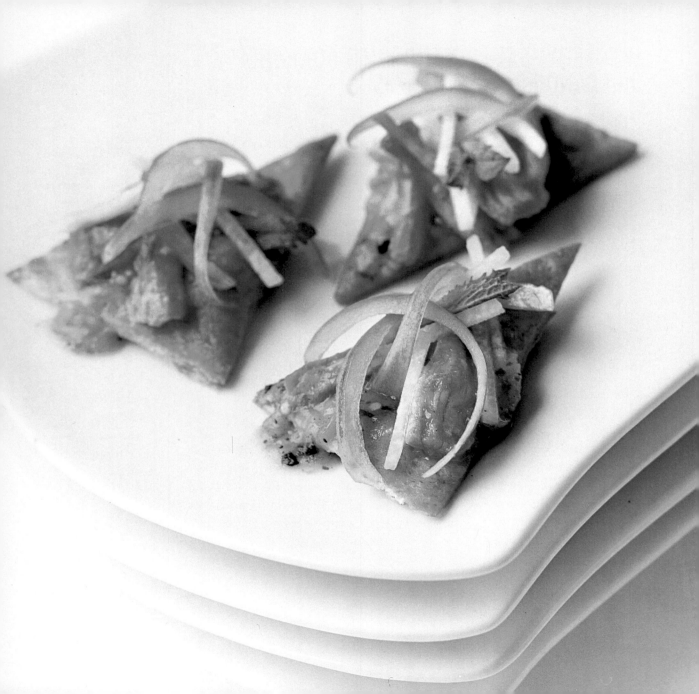

CHILI-BRAISED PORK WITH TOMATILLO SALSA

MAKES 16

When you're in a saucy mood and feel like dancing the rumba, try this amazing shredded pork recipe. I serve it on homemade tortilla chips, but you can use lettuce cups if you want to make this Level One.

Season the pork with salt and pepper. In a braising pan (or stockpot) over medium-high heat, add the 2 tablespoons of the olive oil and the pork. Sear on both sides. Add the onions, peppers, and chilies and allow to caramelize. Add the tomato paste, tomatoes, and chicken broth. Bring to a boil and cover. Reduce the heat to low. Cook until the pork falls apart, about an hour. Remove the pan from the heat. Take out the pork, reserving the liquid in the pan, and allow the pork to cool. Pull the pork into small pieces. Place the pulled pork into a bowl and add 4 to 6 ounces of the liquid.

In a mixing bowl, combine the jicama, red onion, 2 teaspoons of olive oil, and lime juice. Add salt and pepper to taste and set aside. Just before serving, add the mint and mix.

To assemble, scoop a spoonful of Tomatillo Salsa onto each Tortilla Chip, then add a spoonful of the pork mixture and top with the jicama mixture. Serve immediately.

TOMATILLO SALSA

PRO/FATS AND VEGGIES —LEVEL ONE

MAKES ABOUT 3/4 CUP

Preheat the oven to 400 degrees.

Place the tomatillos onto a rimmed baking sheet and drizzle with the olive oil, salt, and pepper. Roast until caramelized and soft, 35 to 45 minutes. Remove from the oven and while still warm, chop until they become the texture of chunky salsa.

TORTILLA CHIPS

LEVEL TWO

Whole-wheat tortillas
Peanut oil

Cut the tortillas into wedges or break into chip-size pieces. Pour the peanut oil into a heavy pot until one-third full. Heat on high until the temperature reaches 375 degrees. Fry the tortillas, a few pieces at a time, until they bubble and float. Remove and drain on paper towels.

LEVEL TWO

1 3-pound pork butt, cut into small chunks
Sea salt and freshly ground black pepper
2 tablespoons plus 2 teaspoons extra-virgin olive oil
1 red onion, medium diced
1 red bell pepper, seeded and medium diced
3 to 4 jalapeño chilies, sliced
2 tablespoons tomato paste
1 cup chopped tomatoes
2 cups chicken broth
1/2 jicama, peeled and finely julienned
1/2 red onion, thinly sliced
2 teaspoons extra-virgin olive oil
Juice from 1/2 lime
1 tablespoon julienned mint leaves
Tomatillo Salsa (recipe follows)
Tortilla Chips (recipe follows)

SALSA
6 tomatillos, peeled, washed, and cut in half
2 tablespoons extra-virgin olive oil
Sea salt and freshly ground black pepper

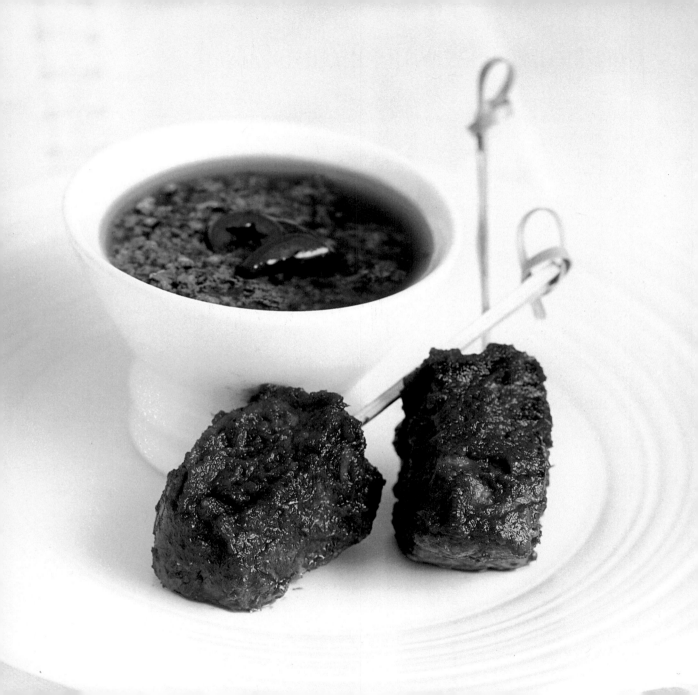

CURRIED LAMB SKEWERS WITH MINT-CILANTRO CHILI PASTE

LEVEL ONE—PRO/FATS
AND VEGGIES

MAKES 16

This mildly spicy lamb is offset perfectly by the freshness of the mint and cilantro. Divine!

In a small bowl, whisk together the curry paste, salt, pepper, oil, lime juice, and curry powder. Transfer to a resealable plastic baggie and add the lamb. Marinate in the refrigerator for 20 to 30 minutes, turning once to evenly coat.

Preheat a grill to medium. Remove the lamb from the marinade and place onto the skewers. Grill until medium rare, 3 to 4 minutes per side. Remove from the heat and serve with the Mint-Cilantro Chili Paste.

2 tablespoons Thai red curry
  paste
Sea salt and freshly ground
  black pepper
1/4 cup extra-virgin olive oil
Juice from 1 lime
2 teaspoons yellow curry
  powder
1 pound lamb loin, cut into
  1-inch cubes
16 wooden skewers, soaked
  in water
Mint-Cilantro Chili Paste
  (recipe follows)

MINT-CILANTRO CHILI PASTE

MAKES ABOUT 1 CUP

Place all the ingredients except the lemon juice into a blender and purée until smooth. Add the lemon juice and pulse to combine. Adjust the seasoning to taste. Refrigerate in an airtight container until ready to use.

ALMOST LEVEL ONE

1/2 bunch fresh cilantro,
  leaves removed
1/2 bunch fresh mint, leaves
  removed
2 tablespoons toasted pine
  nuts
1/4 cup extra-virgin olive oil
Sea salt and freshly ground
  black pepper
Juice from 1/2 lemon

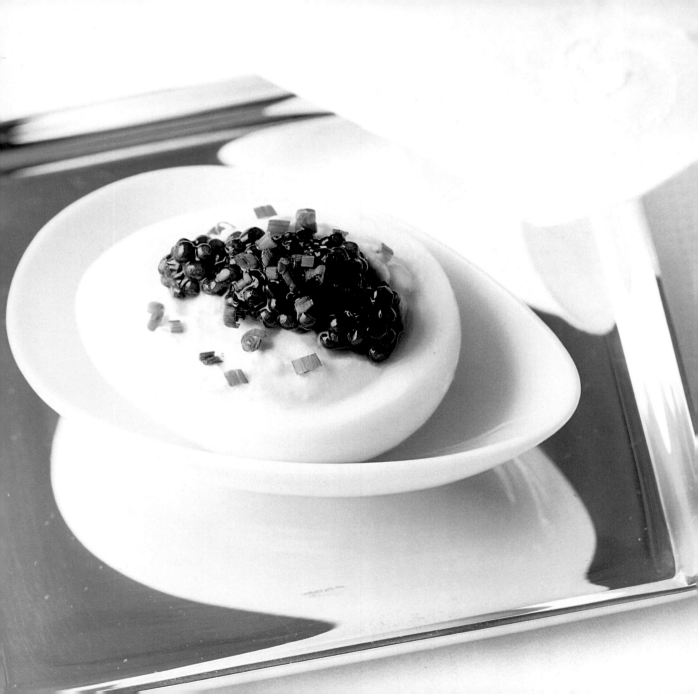

ANGEL EGGS WITH CRÈME FRAÎCHE and CAVIAR

MAKES 16

Why serve deviled eggs when you could have Angel Eggs instead? The addition of caviar and crème fraîche is what makes them so heavenly. Buy the best caviar you can afford.

Slice the eggs in half lengthwise, being careful not to tear the whites. Remove the yolks and press through a fine sieve (or finely chop). In a bowl, mix the egg yolks with the crème fraîche and season with salt and pepper. Spoon a little of the yolk mixture into each egg half and garnish with a dollop of caviar and a sprinkle of chives. Serve immediately.

8 eggs, hard boiled and
   peeled
$1/4$ cup crème fraîche
   (or sour cream)
Sea salt and freshly ground
   black pepper
$1/2$ ounce caviar
2 tablespoons finely minced
   fresh chives

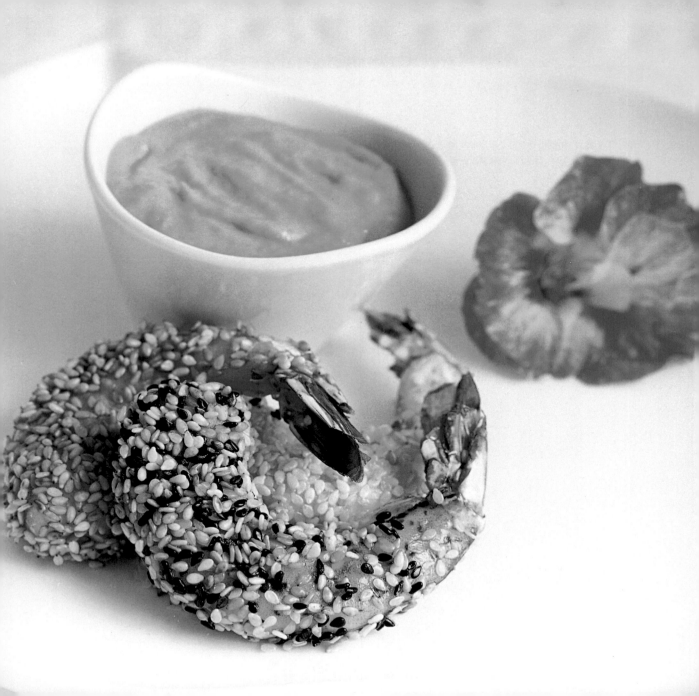

SESAME-CRUSTED SHRIMP WITH MISO DIPPING SAUCE

LEVEL TWO

MAKES 16

Shrimp is a very popular appetizer because it makes a perfect single serving. Here they are crusted in sesame seeds and served with a miso sauce. *You'll* be popular with this recipe.

Preheat the oven to 400 degrees.

Place the shrimp in a mixing bowl and drizzle with olive oil. Season with salt and pepper and coat each shrimp with sesame seeds on both sides.

Place the shrimp onto a rimmed baking sheet and bake for 10 to 15 minutes, until just cooked through. Squeeze lemon juice over shrimp. Serve immediately with the miso sauce.

16 large shrimp, peeled and deveined, tails left on
Extra-virgin olive oil
Sea salt and freshly ground black pepper
3 tablespoons sesame seeds
Juice from 1/2 lemon
Miso Dipping Sauce (recipe follows)

MISO DIPPING SAUCE

ALMOST LEVEL ONE

MAKES 1 CUP

Combine the miso paste, mayonnaise, and lime juice in a small mixing bowl. Season with salt and pepper. Set aside.

1 tablespoon red miso paste
1 cup mayonnaise
Juice from 1/2 lime
Sea salt and freshly ground black pepper

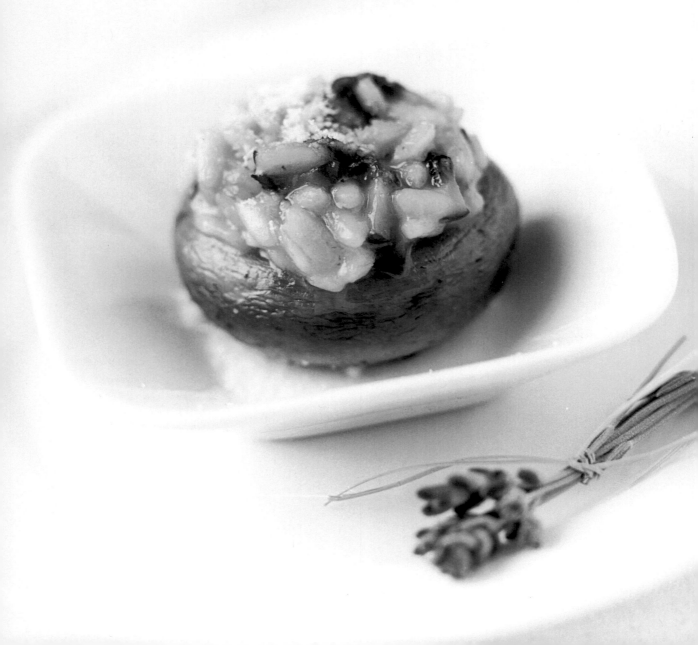

WILD MUSHROOM RISOTTO IN MUSHROOM CAPS

MAKES 16

Risotto is one of my favorite foods. It's creamy and buttery and incredible. It's Level Two, but so worth it. In this recipe I serve a wild mushroom risotto in a mushroom cap for a fantastic passed appetizer. Good luck keeping your spoon out of the pot!

Preheat the oven to 375 degrees.

In an ovenproof dish, place the mushroom caps with the chicken broth and distribute 1 tablespoon butter over the mushrooms. Cover and bake for 25 minutes.

In a saucepan, bring the stock to a boil and reduce to a simmer to keep warm. Place a medium saucepan over medium-high heat. Add 2 tablespoons of the olive oil and the onion. Continuously stir the onion so it does not burn or caramelize. When the onion is soft, after about 5 minutes, add the sliced mushrooms and the remaining tablespoon of oil. Season with salt and pepper. Sauté for 7 to 10 minutes, until the mushrooms are browned and slightly crusty. Add the rice and stir to coat with oil, onions, and mushrooms. Add the wine and allow to reduce until almost dry. Once the wine is reduced, add half of the stock while stirring constantly. As the liquid is absorbed, continue to slowly add the remainder while still stirring. Continue until the risotto is cooked through. Turn off the heat and add the remaining 2 tablespoons of butter and the Parmesan cheese. Stir gently to combine.

Remove the mushrooms from the oven and fill each cap with a spoonful of warm risotto. Garnish with the chervil. Serve immediately.

16 whole mushroom caps, stems removed and discarded
1/4 cup chicken broth
3 tablespoons butter
3 cups mushroom stock or chicken broth
3 tablespoons extra-virgin olive oil
1/2 yellow onion, finely diced
2 cups mixed wild mushrooms, thinly sliced (or regular mushrooms)
Sea salt and freshly ground black pepper
1 cup Arborio rice
1/2 cup white wine
1/2 cup finely grated Parmesan cheese
Fresh chervil leaves, for garnish

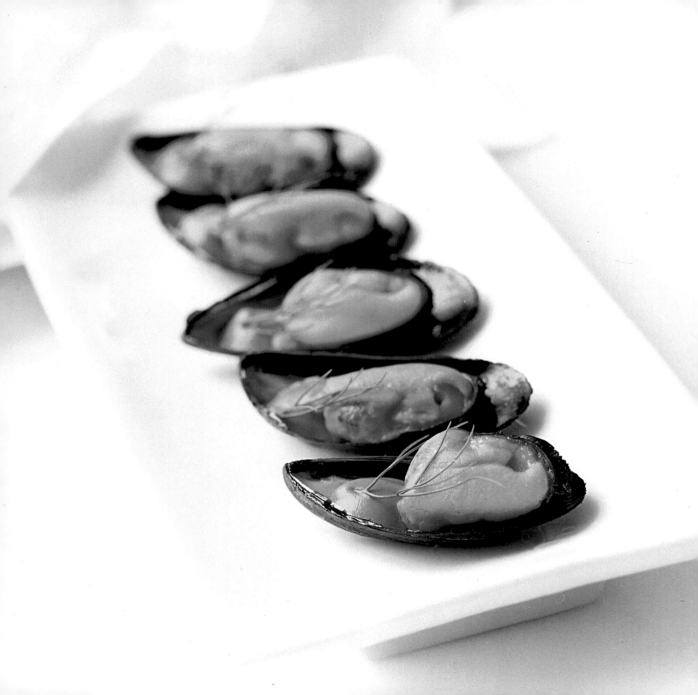

SAFFRON MUSSELS WITH RED PEPPER ROUILLE

MAKES 16

This South of France treat is like having a single bite of bouillabaisse—without the mess!

In a large sauté pan over medium heat, add olive oil to cover bottom of pan. Add the shallots and mussels. Toss to coat with oil. Add the saffron and wine to deglaze the pan. Cover and cook until the mussels open, 3 to 4 minutes. Discard any mussels that do not open. Add the butter and season to taste with salt and pepper. Allow to cool. When cool enough to handle, discard the top half of each shell and serve the mussels on the half shell with a dollop of rouille and one sprig of fresh fennel leaf.

RED PEPPER ROUILLE

MAKES 3/4 CUP

Peel and seed the roasted bell pepper. Purée in a blender with the garlic and olive oil. Mix in the lemon juice. Season to taste with salt and pepper.

LEVEL ONE—PRO/FATS AND VEGGIES

Extra-virgin olive oil
2 tablespoons minced shallots
1 pound mussels (or 16 pieces)
1/4 teaspoon saffron
1 cup white wine
1 tablespoon butter
Sea salt and freshly ground black pepper

FOR GARNISH
1 recipe Red Pepper Rouille (recipe follows)
Fresh fennel leaves

PRO/FATS AND VEGGIES—LEVEL ONE

1 whole red bell pepper, roasted (or 1 jarred roasted red bell pepper)
1 clove garlic, peeled and roasted
1/4 cup extra-virgin olive oil
Juice from 1 lemon
Sea salt and freshly ground black pepper

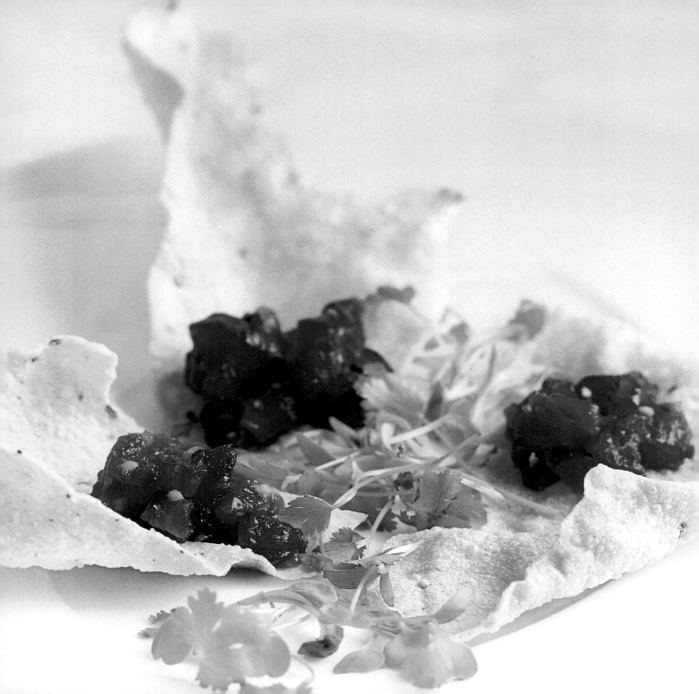

TUNA TARTARE WITH CHILI-GINGER VINAIGRETTE ON PAPPADAM CHIPS

LEVEL TWO

MAKES 16

Pappadam chips are made from Indian lentil flatbread. They are light and crisp and delicious—the perfect accompaniment to this tuna tartare. You can find pappadams at surfasonline.com, or you can use wonton wrappers. For Level One, try Parmesan Crisps (see page 47).

Tear the pappadams into 16 chip-size pieces. Pour peanut oil into a heavy pot until one-third full. Heat on high until the temperature reaches 375 degrees. Fry the pappadams a few pieces at a time until they bubble and float. Remove and drain on paper towels. Set aside.

Clean and dice the tuna. Place in a small mixing bowl with the remaining ingredients, except the cilantro, and mix together. Adjust the seasoning to taste. Spoon the tuna mixture onto a chip, garnish with cilantro, and serve immediately.

4 pieces Indian pappadam flatbread

Peanut oil

1 pound sushi-grade Ahi tuna

1 tablespoon finely minced fresh ginger

1/2 jalapeño or serrano chili, finely minced

2 teaspoons soy sauce

1 teaspoon sesame oil

1 teaspoon rice vinegar

Juice from 1/2 lime

Sea salt and freshly ground black pepper

1 scallion, green ends only, finely chopped

Cilantro leaves, for garnish

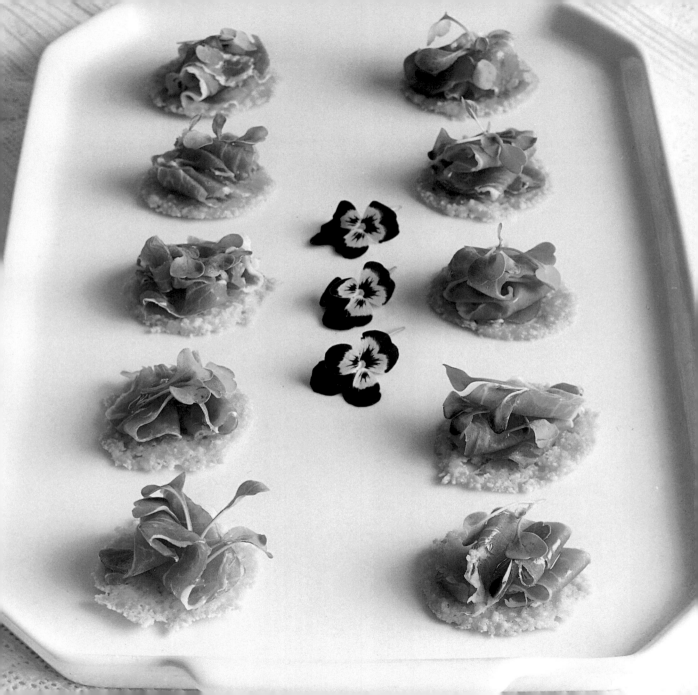

PARMESAN CRISPS WITH PROSCIUTTO and ARUGULA

MAKES 16

LEVEL ONE—PRO/FATS
AND VEGGIES

This is not only simple, it's simply divine! The first time I had this was in Tuscany at my friend Marco's *borgo.* The cracker is made of pure Parmigiano Reggiano (or the best Parmesan you can afford), then topped with prosciutto, arugula, and a drizzle of truffle oil. It's sublime!

16 Parmesan Crisps (recipe
   follows)
8 thin slices prosciutto, cut
   in half across
1 handful baby arugula
Truffle oil (or extra-virgin
   olive oil)
Freshly ground black pepper

Place a piece of prosciutto, a leaf of arugula, and a drizzle of truffle oil on each Parmesan crisp. Season with freshly ground pepper.

PARMESAN CRISPS

MAKES 16 CRISPS

LEVEL ONE—PRO/FATS

½ cup finely shredded
   Parmigiano Reggiano
   cheese

Preheat the oven to 350 degrees.

Line a baking sheet with parchment paper (or a Silpat nonstick mat). Sprinkle the cheese into 3-inch circles, making several mini "pancakes." Place into the oven for about 5 minutes, until just golden.

Remove from the oven and let cool slightly.

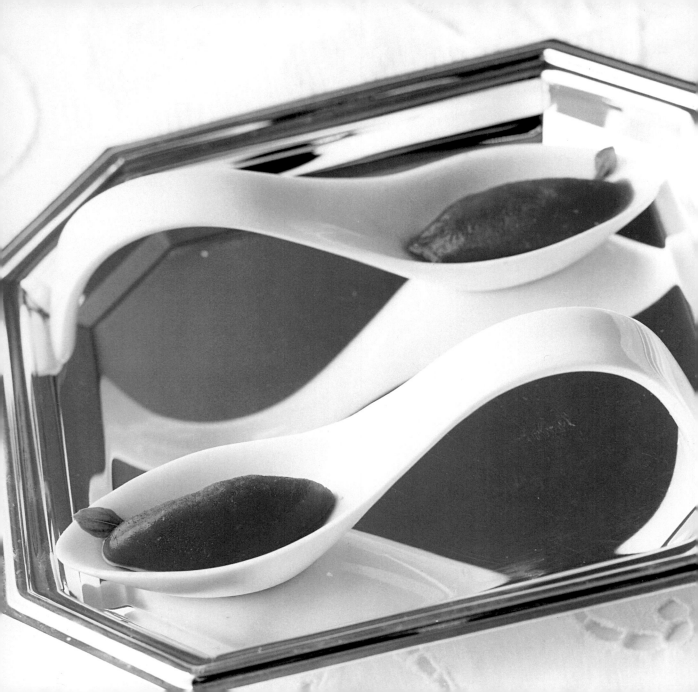

SPICY TOMATO SORBET WITH CRACKED BLACK PEPPER AND BASIL

SERVES 10

Sorbet as an appetizer? Made from tomatoes? You bet. This unique taste is like nothing you've ever had before, and it will wow your guests. As a passed appetizer I serve it on pretty spoons. At the table you could use a very small ice-cream dish or even a demitasse cup.

In a small saucepan over medium heat, add the olive oil, garlic, and jalapeño. Allow to brown and add the tomatoes. Cook until caramelized, about 7 minutes, stirring occasionally. Deglaze with the white wine and season with salt and pepper. Once the wine has reduced by half, add ¼ cup water and one basil sprig, including the stem. Cook until the tomatoes are broken down and soft, 10 to 15 minutes. Discard the basil sprig and transfer the tomato mixture to a blender. (Always allow hot items to cool before blending. Steam can cause the blender lid to pop off and spray hot liquid.) Purée on high until smooth, 3 to 4 minutes. Strain through a medium sieve. Adjust the seasonings with salt and pepper. Place into the refrigerator and chill.

Freeze the tomato mixture in an ice-cream maker according to the manufacturer's instructions. Store in an airtight container in the freezer until ready to serve.

Serve small bites of the sorbet in tablespoons or Asian soup spoons. Garnish with cracked black pepper and fresh basil.

2 tablespoons extra-virgin
   olive oil
1 clove garlic, peeled
½ jalapeño chili, seeds
   removed, small diced
6 to 8 Roma tomatoes, cut
   into small chunks
¼ cup white wine
Sea salt and freshly ground
   black pepper
1 sprig fresh basil

FOR GARNISH
Cracked black pepper
10 fresh basil leaves,
   finely julienned

49

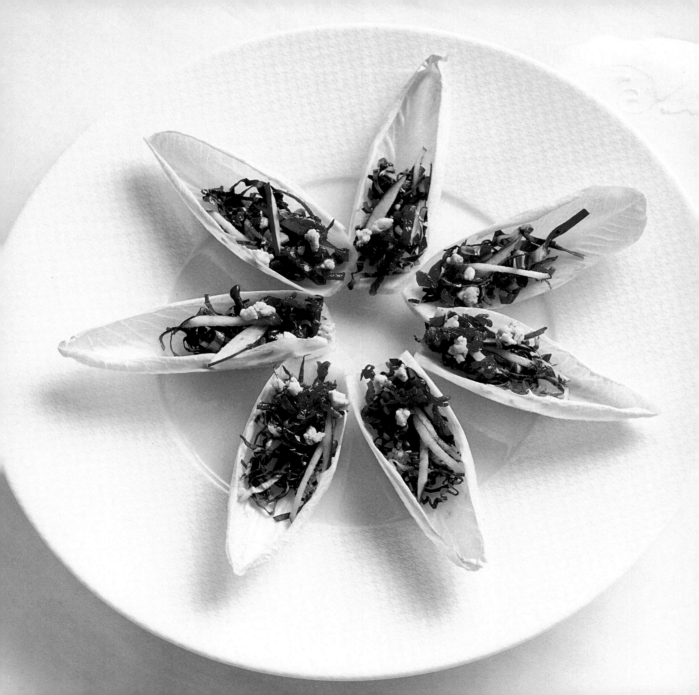

ENDIVE SPEARS WITH APPLE, PROSCIUTTO, and GORGONZOLA

MAKES 16

In a word: fabulous!

In a medium-size sauté pan, add olive oil to cover the bottom of the pan and heat on medium high. Add the prosciutto and cook until crisp. Remove from the oil and drain on paper towels.

To assemble, lay endive spears on a work surface and top each spear with small amounts of spinach, radicchio, apple, prosciutto, and a sprinkling of cheese. Season with salt and pepper. Serve immediately.

Extra-virgin olive oil
4 slices prosciutto, julienned
16 endive spears, washed
1 cup baby spinach leaves, julienned
1 head radicchio, julienned
1 Fuji or Gala apple, julienned (omit for Level One)
4 ounces Gorgonzola cheese, cut into small pieces
Sea salt and freshly ground black pepper

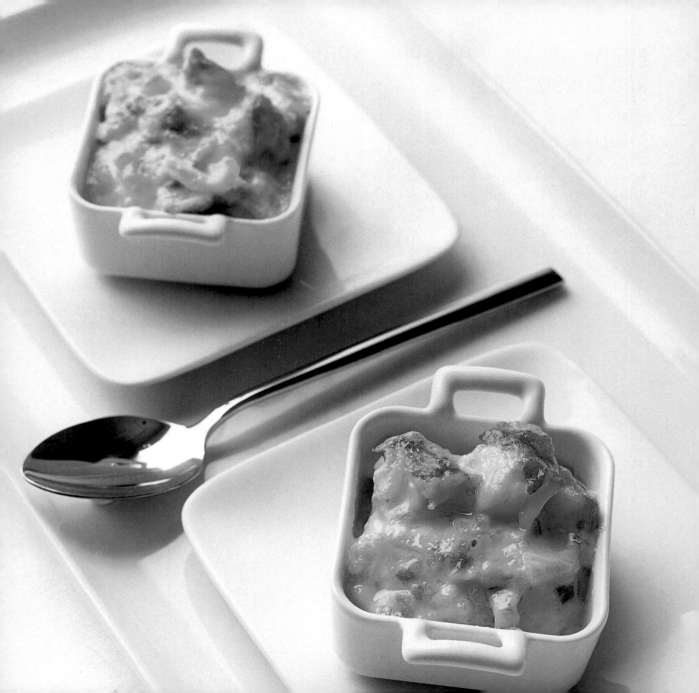

LOBSTER THERMIDOR

SERVES 12

Lobster Thermidor is a classic baked lobster dish. It's traditionally served in lobster shells, but as a first course you may serve it in small ramekins. I also love to serve it as a passed appetizer, as little bites of heaven lined up in Asian spoons. My guests love this one.

To make the lobster, chop the lobster meat into ¼-inch pieces. Place a large sauté pan over medium heat and add 1 tablespoon olive oil, the butter, celery, shallots, and mushrooms. Sauté until soft and caramelized, about 5 minutes. Add the lobster and toss just until warm, then season with salt and pepper. Remove from the heat and set aside.

To make the sauce, in a metal or glass bowl set over a pot of water or the top of a double boiler, combine the egg yolks, lemon juice, and 2 teaspoons water over medium heat. Continuously whisk the mixture. Cook until the eggs are fluffy but not scrambled. Once the eggs are light and fluffy, incorporate butter one piece at a time with a whisk, allowing it to cook into the sauce. Don't rush it, or the sauce will break. The sauce should have the consistency of a thin mayonnaise. Remove from the heat, keeping the sauce warm. Season to taste with salt and pepper. Add the cayenne and Tabasco.

Preheat the broiler.

In a separate bowl, combine the lobster mixture with 1 cup of the sauce and the mayonnaise. Place into individual ovenproof dishes (or one shallow casserole dish), sprinkle with Parmesan cheese, and broil until bubbly and golden brown, about 5 minutes. Serve individual ramekins immediately. If serving as a passed appetizer, spoon bites onto Asian soup spoons, lined up on a tray.

FOR THE LOBSTER
1 whole lobster, 1½ to
  2 pounds, cooked and
  cleaned
Extra-virgin olive oil
1 tablespoon butter
¼ cup finely diced celery
¼ cup finely diced shallots
  or onion
¼ cup finely diced
  mushrooms
Sea salt and freshly ground
  black pepper

FOR THE SAUCE
3 egg yolks
Juice from ½ lemon
1 cup (2 sticks) butter, cut
  into pieces
Sea salt and freshly ground
  black pepper
1 pinch cayenne pepper
1 dash Tabasco sauce

¼ cup mayonnaise
Parmesan cheese, for garnish

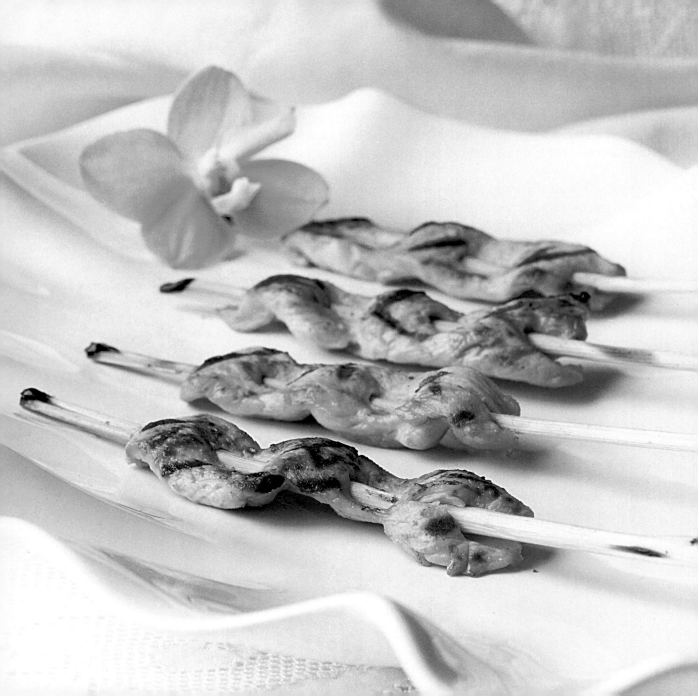

MISO CHICKEN SKEWERS

MAKES 16

Many people are intimidated by Asian ingredients, but rice vinegar and miso paste are readily available and easy to work with. These chicken skewers are delicious and a nice change from your typical satay. For an exotic presentation, use lemongrass stalks as skewers.

For the marinade, mix together the vinegar, miso paste, and olive oil and season with salt and pepper. Place the chicken strips into the marinade and refrigerate for 30 minutes.

Preheat the grill. Secure 1 chicken strip per skewer and grill over medium heat until cooked through, about 3 minutes per side. Serve immediately.

1 tablespoon rice vinegar

2 tablespoons miso paste

1 tablespoon extra-virgin olive oil

Sea salt and freshly ground black pepper

2 boneless, skinless chicken breasts, cut into small strips

16 wooden skewers, soaked in water (or lemongrass stalks)

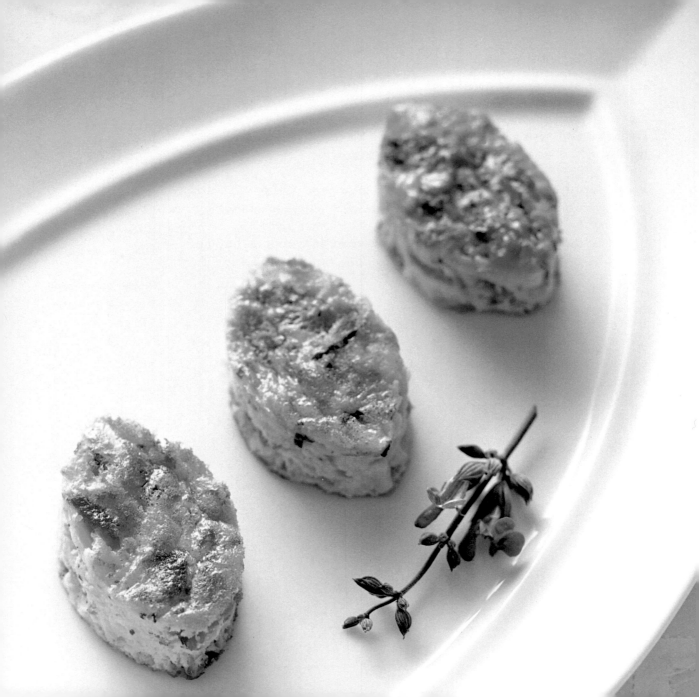

SOMER FRITTATA

SERVES 8

Frittatas are easy and delicious. Cut them into interesting shapes and serve warm or at room temperature.

Preheat the oven to 325 degrees.

Butter a glass 8 x 8-inch baking dish. In a medium sauté pan over medium heat, add the olive oil, onions, and pancetta. Sauté until the pancetta is rendered of fat and onions are caramelized, about 10 minutes. Remove from the heat, drain excess fat, and allow to cool.

In a mixing bowl, beat the eggs and add the cream, cheeses, herbs, and onion-pancetta mixture. Season with salt and pepper. Pour into the baking dish and bake until set, 35 to 40 minutes. Remove from the oven and cut into bite-size pieces. Serve immediately.

1 tablespoon butter
1 tablespoon extra-virgin
  olive oil
1 cup diced onions
1 cup diced pancetta
  (or bacon)
6 eggs
$1/4$ cup heavy cream
$3/4$ cup grated soft cheese
  (Fontina or Asiago)
$1/2$ cup finely grated
  Parmesan cheese
2 tablespoons julienned
  fresh basil
2 tablespoons finely
  chopped fresh chives
1 tablespoon chopped fresh
  flat-leaf parsley
Sea salt and freshly ground
  black pepper

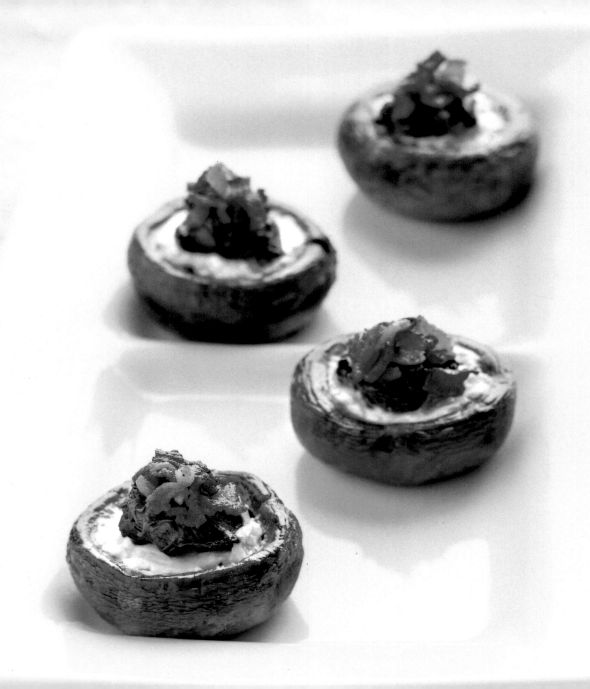

ROASTED MUSHROOMS WITH SPINACH, CHEESE, AND PANCETTA

MAKES 16

The mushroom cap is a perfect vegetable "spoon"—great for when you don't want added carbs. This is filled with wonderful tastes of goat cheese, spinach, and pancetta.

Preheat the oven to 350 degrees.

Place the mushrooms, stem side up, into a baking dish. Season with salt and pepper and place a small piece of butter into the center of each cap. Bake until cooked through, about 20 minutes. While the mushrooms are roasting, in a sauté pan over medium heat, add ½ tablespoon of the olive oil and the spinach. Sauté until the spinach is wilted. Set aside.

In another sauté pan over medium heat, use the remaining ½ tablespoon of olive oil to cook the onions and pancetta until the pancetta is rendered of fat and the onions are slightly caramelized. Drain excess fat and set aside.

When the mushrooms are cooked, remove them from the oven. When cool enough to handle, fill each one with a spoonful of goat cheese, then top with spinach and the pancetta mixture. Serve immediately.

16 mushroom caps, washed, stems removed
Sea salt and freshly ground black pepper
2 tablespoons butter, cut into small pieces
1 tablespoon extra-virgin olive oil
1 pound fresh spinach, washed and stemmed
½ cup small-diced onion
½ cup small-diced pancetta (or bacon)
1 cup fresh goat cheese

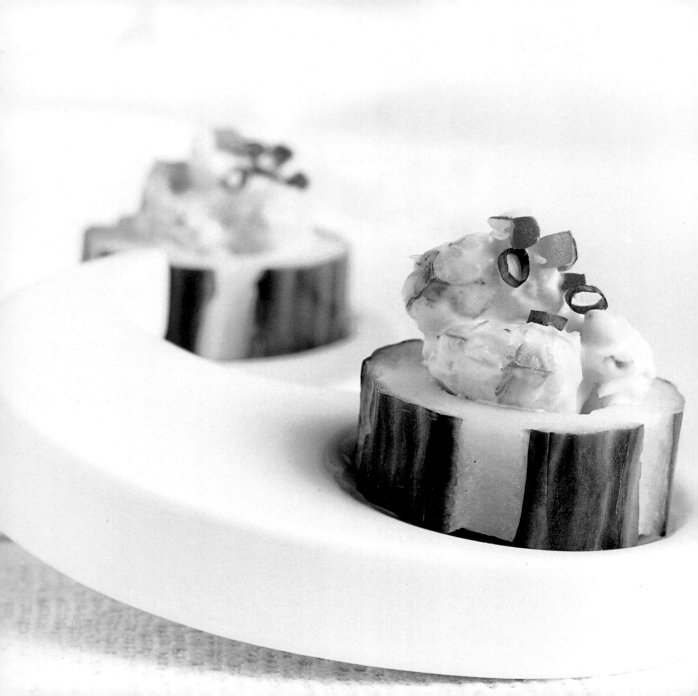

ROCK SHRIMP SALAD ON CUCUMBER ROUNDS

MAKES 16

Rock shrimp adds a whole different flavor to shrimp salad. The taste is like lobster: buttery and delicious. I serve this on chunky cucumber rounds that have been slightly scooped out.

In a medium sauté pan over medium heat, add the olive oil and garlic. As the garlic becomes golden brown, add the shrimp and cook until just done, 3 to 4 minutes. Remove from the heat and chill.

In a mixing bowl, combine the mayonnaise, sour cream, bell pepper, onion, scallions, and a dash of Tabasco. Chop half the shrimp and leave the other half whole, then add all the shrimp to the salad ingredients and mix well. Adjust the seasoning with salt, pepper, and lemon juice. Set aside.

Peel the cucumber in 4 strips lengthwise to create a wide scoring effect, then slice into ½-inch rounds. Carefully scoop out some of the seeds to create a small indentation (without scooping all the way through) to cradle the filling. Fill each cucumber slice with a scoop of shrimp salad and serve immediately.

---

1 tablespoon extra-virgin olive oil

1 clove garlic, smashed

½ pound rock shrimp, cleaned

½ cup mayonnaise

¼ cup sour cream

½ red bell pepper, seeded and finely diced

½ red onion, finely diced

2 scallions, finely diced

Tabasco sauce

Sea salt and freshly ground black pepper

Juice from 1 lemon

1 cucumber

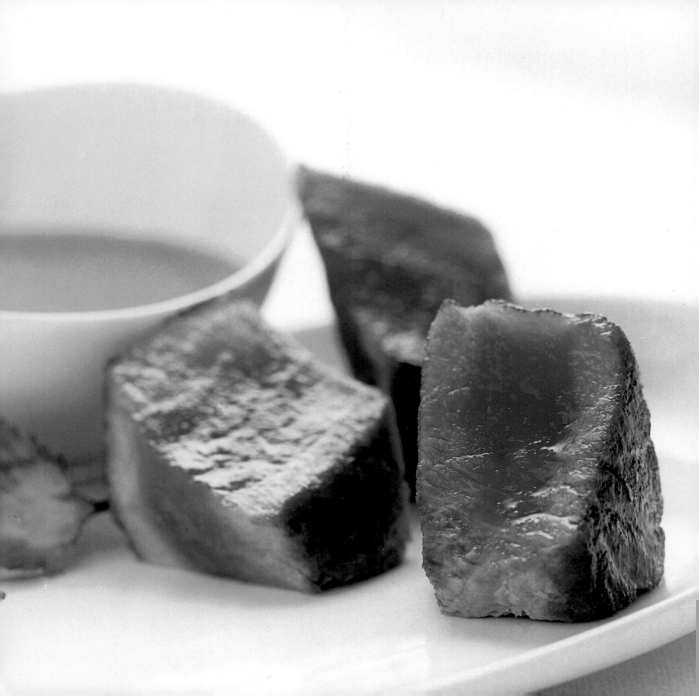

SEARED TUNA WITH CILANTRO-ORANGE SAUCE

LEVEL ONE—PRO/FATS
AND VEGGIES

MAKES 16

Although I am not a huge fish eater, I absolutely love fresh Ahi tuna. In this recipe I sear it, then serve it with a snappy cilantro-orange sauce with scallions and lime. Very tasty.

Season the tuna with salt and pepper. Heat a light coating of olive oil in a sauté pan over medium-high heat, then sear the tuna on all sides until golden brown on the outside but rare in the center. Remove from the heat and drizzle with soy sauce and lime juice. Place on a platter and serve with Cilantro-Orange Sauce.

8 ounces Ahi tuna, cut into
   bite-size cubes
Sea salt and freshly ground
   black pepper
Extra-virgin olive oil
Dash of soy sauce
Juice from $1/2$ lime
Cilantro-Orange Sauce
   (recipe follows)

CILANTRO-ORANGE SAUCE

LEVEL TWO

MAKES 1 CUP

Combine all the ingredients in a blender and purée until smooth. Set aside.

$1/2$ cup orange juice
1 tablespoon miso paste
2 tablespoons chopped
   fresh cilantro
2 tablespoons chopped
   scallions
Juice from 1 lime
$1/2$ cup extra-virgin olive oil

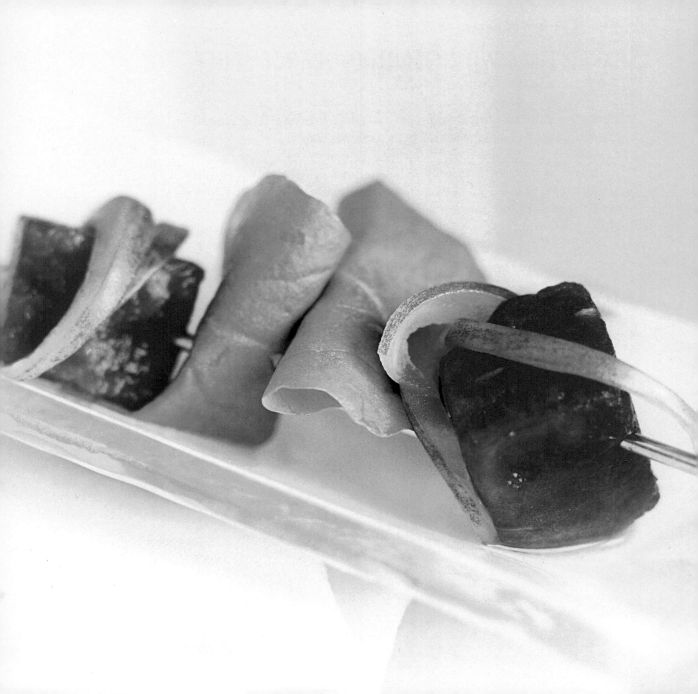

SUMMER SALAD ON A SKEWER

MAKES 16

This unique salad is simply smashing! The sweetness of the watermelon with the slightly bitter watercress creates a stunning combination. I had a Cuban party and served this as a salad course on a bed of watercress. Or you can thread it onto a skewer for a fabulous passed appetizer.

Place the sliced onion into a bowl and add the vinegar, SomerSweet, salt, and pepper. Set aside for at least 15 minutes to pickle the onions.

Pass the raspberries through a fine sieve into a mixing bowl. Discard the seeds and pulp. Add the watermelon to the raspberries and season with salt and pepper. Add the pickled onions and toss gently to combine.

To assemble, place 1 large watercress leaf onto a skewer followed by a watermelon chunk. Continue until all skewers are complete. Arrange on a platter and sprinkle with the remaining pickled onions. Drizzle with the olive oil and serve immediately.

1 red onion, thinly sliced

1/4 cup champagne vinegar

1/4 teaspoon SomerSweet (or 1 teaspoon sugar)

Sea salt and freshly ground black pepper

1/4 cup raspberries

2 cups of 3/4-inch cubes of watermelon

1 bunch watercress, cleaned and picked over

1 tablespoon extra-virgin olive oil

16 wooden skewers

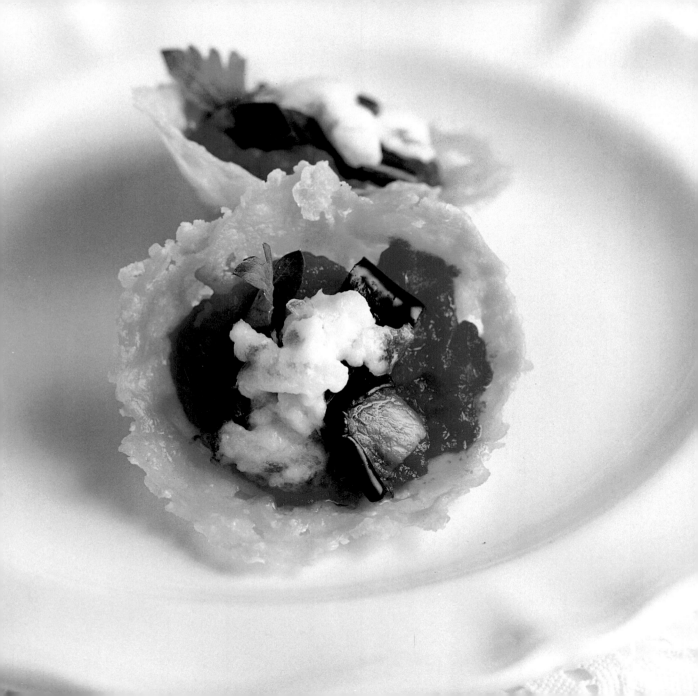

MELTED BURRATA CHEESE WITH ROASTED EGGPLANT AND BASIL IN PARMESAN CUPS

MAKES 16

Burrata is a fabulous soft Italian cheese. It melts beautifully and tastes great paired with roasted eggplant. Add the crunch of a Parmesan cup and it's a winner.

To make the Parmesan cups, follow the directions for Parmesan Crisps (see page 47); but when they come out of the oven, form them into cups by placing them over the bottoms of small glasses. Set aside.

Preheat the oven to 350 degrees.

Quarter the eggplants lengthwise into spears. Drizzle with olive oil, season with salt and pepper, and place on a baking sheet. Roast until soft, 20 to 25 minutes. Remove from the oven. When cool enough to handle, cut into medium dice.

On another baking sheet, create 16 small piles of eggplant, about 2 pieces of eggplant per pile. Top each with about ½ tablespoon of the cheese. Bake for about 5 minutes, or until the cheese melts.

To assemble, place a dollop of tomato sauce into each Parmesan cup, then use a spatula to scrape the eggplant and cheese into the cup. Garnish with the basil and serve immediately.

16 Parmesan cups
  (see below)
3 Japanese eggplants
Extra-virgin olive oil
Sea salt and freshly ground
  black pepper
1 cup fresh Burrata cheese
  (or mozzarella)
½ cup tomato sauce,
  warmed
2 tablespoons julienned
  basil, for garnish

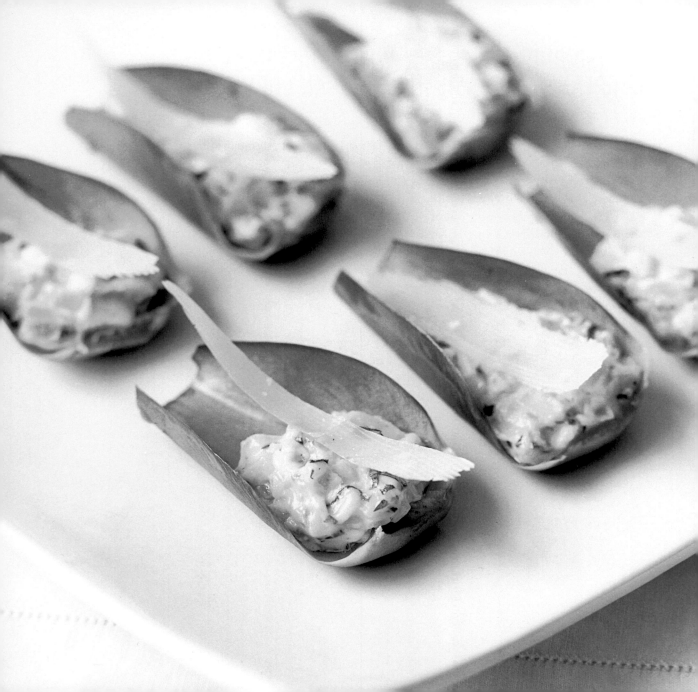

ARTICHOKE LEAVES WITH TARRAGON AÏOLI and SHAVED PARMESAN

MAKES 16

Artichokes are one of my favorite foods. For casual entertaining you can serve a whole artichoke and place a bowl for the discarded leaves in the center of the table. Here's a way to serve artichokes as a passed hors d'oeuvre with a bit of fanfare. The "aïoli" is a snap to make.

Finely chop the artichoke hearts and mix with the mayonnaise, garlic, tarragon, lemon juice, salt, and pepper. Select 16 perfect artichoke leaves and arrange on a tray. (The outside leaves will be more sturdy to hold the filling.) Place a dollop of the aïoli filling on each leaf. Garnish with a slice of shaved Parmesan cheese and serve immediately.

2 whole artichokes, steamed,
　　leaves removed and hearts
　　cleaned and set aside
1 cup mayonnaise
1 teaspoon finely chopped
　　garlic
2 tablespoons chopped fresh
　　tarragon
Juice from 1/2 lemon
Sea salt and freshly ground
　　black pepper
Shaved Parmesan, for garnish

69

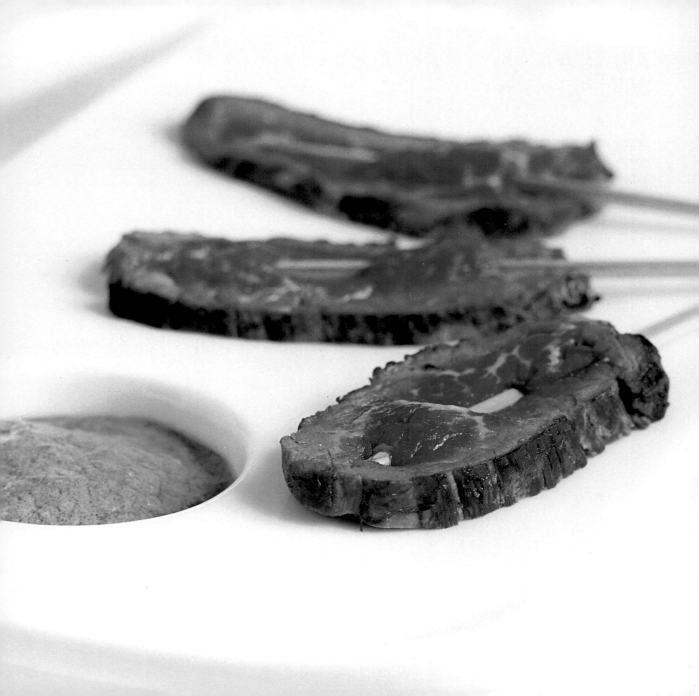

SEARED BEEF WITH LIME-CHILI-MINT DIPPING SAUCE

MAKES 16

This bright green dipping sauce not only looks great; its taste will drive you wild.

Preheat the oven to 400 degrees.

In a medium sauté pan over high heat, add 1 tablespoon of the olive oil. Season the beef with salt and pepper and sear all over until nicely browned, about 4 minutes. Remove from the heat and set aside.

To make the dipping sauce, in a blender combine the mint leaves with the serrano chili. Add the remaining olive oil slowly and purée to make a smooth paste. Add the lime juice and season with salt and pepper.

Cut the beef on the diagonal into ¼-inch slices. Thread each slice onto a skewer. When ready to serve, place the skewers into an ovenproof pan and drizzle with the soy sauce and olive oil. Heat in the oven for 3 to 4 minutes. Serve immediately with the dipping sauce.

½ cup extra-virgin olive oil, plus more for drizzling
½-pound piece of beef tenderloin (or your favorite cut of meat)
Sea salt and freshly ground black pepper
1 cup fresh mint leaves
1 serrano chili, chopped
Juice from 1 lime
2 tablespoons light soy sauce
16 wooden skewers, soaked in water

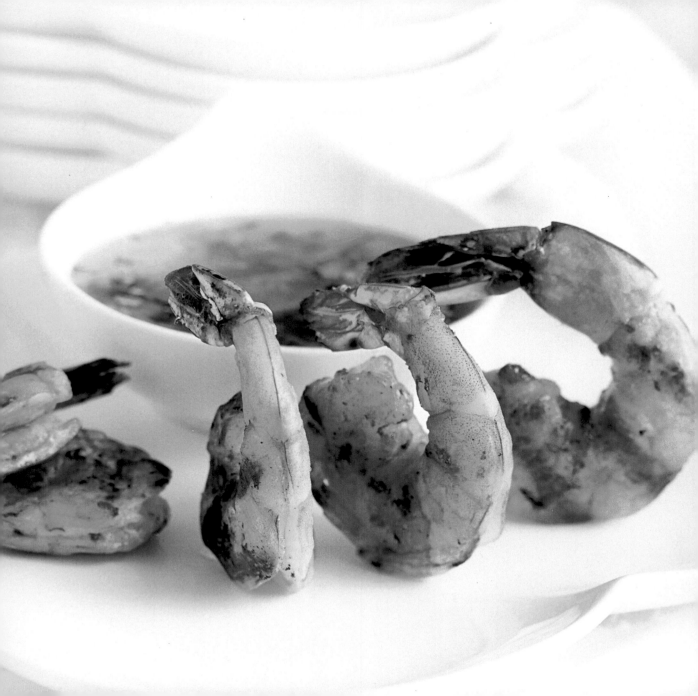

SWEET SHRIMP WITH HOT GREEN CHUTNEY

MAKES 16

This Asian-influenced shrimp is combined with a knockout spicy and sweet chutney. A great alternative to cocktail sauce.

To make the chutney, in a medium saucepan over medium heat, add the olive oil, onions, and ginger. Cook until the onions are soft, 5 to 6 minutes, stirring occasionally. Add the vinegar and SomerSweet. Simmer for 2 minutes. Remove from the heat and allow to cool. When cool, add the jalapeño, serrano, and herbs. Adjust the seasoning with salt and pepper. Set aside to serve with the shrimp.

To make the shrimp, season the shrimp with salt and pepper. In a medium sauté pan over medium heat, add a tablespoon of olive oil. Add the shrimp, gently searing on both sides. Add the wine. Reduce the heat and cover. Cook until the shrimp are just cooked through, about 3 minutes, depending upon their size. Remove from the heat, and place the shrimp onto a plate.

Serve the shrimp with the chutney dipping sauce.

FOR THE CHUTNEY
1 tablespoon extra-virgin
 olive oil
1/2 yellow onion, finely diced
2 tablespoons finely minced
 fresh ginger
1/4 cup rice vinegar
1/2 teaspoon SomerSweet
 (or 2 teaspoons sugar)
1 red jalapeño, finely minced
1 serrano chili, finely minced
1/2 cup chopped fresh cilantro
1/4 cup chopped fresh basil
1/4 cup chopped fresh mint
Sea salt and freshly ground
 black pepper

FOR THE SHRIMP
16 large raw shrimp, peeled
 and deveined, tail left on
Sea salt and freshly ground
 black pepper
Extra-virgin olive oil
2 cups white wine

Accessories Guide

Lobster Bisque Cappuccino: Imported porcelain "White Espresso" cup and saucer by BIA /Cordon Bleu available at Sur La Table, 161 West Colorado Blvd., Pasadena, CA 91105, 626-844-2917. For the store nearest you, call 800-243-0852 or visit www.surlatable.com. Imported rectangular earthenware platter available exclusively at Williams-Sonoma, 142 South Lake Blvd., Pasadena, CA 91101, 626-795-5045. For the store nearest you, call 800-541-1262 or visit www.williams-sonoma.com. Porcelain condiment spoon available at Crate & Barrel, 75 West Colorado Blvd., Pasadena, CA 91105, 626-683-8000. For the store nearest you, call 800-323-5461 or visit www.crateandbarrel.com. Imported French damask linen available at Maison Midi, 148 South La Brea, Los Angeles, CA 90036, 323-935-3157.

Radicchio Cups with Curried Chicken: Square ceramic "wave" plate available at Crate & Barrel, 75 West Colorado Blvd., Pasadena, CA 91105, 626-683-8000. For the store nearest you, call 800-323-5461 or visit www.crateandbarrel.com. Antique crochet and lace linen tablecloth (asst.) available at Bountiful Harvest, 1335 Abbot Kinney Blvd., Venice, CA 90291, 310-450-3620.

Mini Burgers with Gorgonzola and Caramelized Onions: "Quartet" dinner plate available at Crate & Barrel, 75 West Colorado Blvd., Pasadena, CA 91105, 626-683-8000. For the store nearest you, call 800-323-5461 or visit www.crateandbarrel.com. Vintage crochet and cotton linens (asst.) available at Bountiful Harvest, 1335 Abbot Kinney Blvd., Venice, CA 90291, 310-450-3620.

Grilled Scallops Wrapped in Prosciutto with Basil-Parsley Pistou: Square appetizer plate available exclusively at Crate & Barrel, 75 West Colorado Blvd., Pasadena, CA 91105, 626-683-8000. For the store nearest you, call 800-323-5461 or visit www.crateandbarrel.com. Antique linen from Suzanne's private collection. Herbs by Country Fresh Herbs, 18211 Emelita Street, Tarzana, CA 91356, 818-345-8810.

Mini Lettuce Cups with Minced Duck: Sushi plate (8.5") available at Sur La Table, 161 West Colorado Blvd., Pasadena, CA 91105, 626-844-2917. Linens from Suzanne's private collection.

Beef Bourguigorne Brochettes: "Horizon" medium-sized oval plate available exclusively at Crate & Barrel, 75 West Colorado Blvd., Pasadena, CA 91105, 626-683-8000. For the store nearest you, call 800-323-5461 or visit www.crateandbarrel.com. Antique Battenburg lace and linen tablecloth (asst.) available at Bountiful Harvest, 1335 Abbot Kinney Blvd., Venice, CA 90291, 310-450-3620. Herbs by Country Fresh Herbs, 18211 Emelita Street, Tarzana, CA 91356, 818-345-8810.

Artichoke Bottoms with Dungeness Crab Salad: Square white dish (3" x 3") and washable hemstitch linen tablecloth (exclusively) available at Crate & Barrel, 75 West Colorado Blvd., Pasadena, CA 91105, 626-683-8000. For the store nearest you, call 800-323-5461 or visit www.crateandbarrel.com.

Clams Gratin with Pancetta and Arugula: Jelly roll pan available at Sur La Table, 161 West Colorado Blvd., Pasadena, CA 91105, 626-844-2917. Stained-glass surface available at Stained Glass Supply, 2104 Colorado Blvd., Eagle Rock, CA 90041, 323-254-4361.

Whole-Wheat Crostini with Goat Cheese and Candied Tomato Relish: Small square plate available at Crate & Barrel, 75 West Colorado Blvd., Pasadena, CA 91105, 626-683-8000. For the store nearest you, call 800-323-5461 or visit www.crateandbarrel.com. Antique Battenburg lace tablecloth (asst.) available at Bountiful Harvest, 1335 Abbot Kinney Blvd., Venice, CA 90291, 310-450-3620.

Chili-Braised Pork with Tomatillo Salsa: "Wave Pit Triangle" plate available at Crate & Barrel, 75 West Colorado Blvd., Pasadena, CA 91105, 626-683-8000. For the store nearest you, call 800-323-5461 or visit www.crateandbarrel.com. Stained-glass surface available at Stained Glass Supply, 2104 Colorado Blvd., Eagle Rock, CA 90041, 323-254-4361. Herbs by Country Fresh Herbs, 18211 Emelita Street, Tarzana, CA 91356, 818-345-8810.

Curried Lamb Skewers with Mint-Cilantro Chili Paste: Jasper Conran 7-inch "Swirl Plate" by Wedgwood available at Geary's of Beverly Hills, 351 North Beverly Drive, Beverly Hills, CA 90210, 310-273-4741 or 800-793-6670, www.gearys.com. "Footed Sauce" 1.5 oz pipkin available exclusively at Crate & Barrel, 75 West Colorado Blvd., Pasadena, CA 91105, 626-683-8000. For the store nearest you, call 800-323-5461 or visit www.crateandbarrel.com. Pull-stitch lace linen napkin available at Buyers Services, 379 South Robertson, Beverly Hills, CA 90211, 310-273-8526 or 800-551-8710.

Angel Eggs with Crème Fraîche and Caviar: Silver coaster (tray) by Ercuis Silver available at Buyers Services, 379 South Robertson, Beverly Hills, CA 90211, 310-273-8526 or 800-551-8710. "Quenell" dish forme point sans décor by Raynaud available at Lucy Zahran, 189 Grove Drive, Los Angeles, CA 90036, 310-273-1338 or 800-828-1333. Imported "Round Scroll Appliqué" linen napkin available at Geary's of Beverly Hills, 351 North Beverly Drive, Beverly Hills, CA 90210, 310-273-4741 or 800-793-6670, www.gearys.com.

Sesame-Crusted Shrimp with Miso Dipping Sauce: Richard Ginori "Didalo" plate and "Octagonal Scroll Border" napkin available at Geary's of Beverly Hills, 351 North Beverly Drive, Beverly Hills, CA 90210, 310-273-4741 or 800-793-6670, www.gearys.com. "Cocoon" bowl imported by Williams-Sonoma, 142 South Lake Blvd., Pasadena, CA 91101, 626-795-5045. For the store nearest you, call 800-541-1262 or visit www.williams-sonoma.com. Herbs by Country Fresh Herbs, 18211 Emelita Street, Tarzana, CA 91356, 818-345-8810.

Wild Mushroom Risotto in Mushroom Caps: BIA/Cordon Bleu salad plate available at Surfas, 310-559-4770, www.surfasonline.com. "Quartet" square ramekin imported from Germany by Crate & Barrel, 75 West Colorado Blvd., Pasadena, CA 91105, 626-683-8000. For the store nearest you, call 800-323-5461 or visit www.crateandbarrel.com. Antique damask with Greek key design (asst.) available at Bountiful Harvest, 1335 Abbot Kinney Blvd., Venice, CA 90291, 310-450-3620. Herbs by Country Fresh Herbs, 18211 Emelita Street, Tarzana, CA 91356, 818-345-8810.

Saffron Mussels with Red Pepper Rouille: Imported porcelain BIA/Cordon Bleu platter available at Surfas, 310-559-4770, www.surfasonline.com. Imported linen "Round Scroll Appliqué" napkin available at Geary's of Beverly Hills, 351 North Beverly Drive, Beverly Hills, CA 90210, 310-273-4741 or 800-793-6670, www.gearys.com.

Tuna Tartare with Chili-Ginger Vinaigrette on Pappadam Chips: "Fish Center" platter by Raynaud available at Lucy Zahran, 189 Grove Drive, Los Angeles, CA 90036, 310-273-1338 or 800-828-1333. Imported jacquard napkin available exclusively at Maison Midi, 148 South La Brea, Los Angeles, CA 90036, 323-935-

3157. Herbs by Country Fresh Herbs, 18211 Emelita Street, Tarzana, CA 91356, 818-345-8810.

Parmesan Crisps with Proscuitto and Arugula: Rectangular (14" x 8"), two-handled porcelain platter available exclusively at Sur La Table, 161 West Colorado Blvd., Pasadena, CA 91105, 626-844-2917. For the store nearest you, call 800-243-0852 or visit www.surlatable.com. Antique open-cut eyelet tablecloth (asst.) available at Bountiful Harvest, 1335 Abbot Kinney Blvd., Venice, CA 90291, 310-450-3620. Pansies by Country Fresh Herbs, 18211 Emelita Street, Tarzana, CA 91356, 818-345-8810.

Spicy Tomato Sorbet with Cracked Black Pepper and Basil: Octagonal silver tray available at Buyers Services, 379 South Robertson, Beverly Hills, CA 90211, 310-273-8526 or 800-551-8710. Porcelain spoons by Thomas Keller for Raynaud available at De Vine Corporation, 732-751-0500, www.devinecorp.net. Antique pull-stitch linen tablecloth (asst.) available at Bountiful Harvest, 1335 Abbot Kinney Blvd., Venice, CA 90291, 310-450-3620. Herbs by Country Fresh Herbs, 18211 Emelita Street, Tarzana, CA 91356. 818-345-8810.

Endive Spears with Apple, Proscuitto, and Gorgonzola: Porcelain "Cheques" service plate by Thomas Keller for Raynaud available at De Vine Corporation, 732-751-0500, www.devinecorp.net. "Oblong Wave" linen napkin by George Henry available at Geary's of Beverly Hills, 351 North Beverly Drive, Beverly Hills, CA 90210, 310-273-4741 or 800-793-6670, www.gearys.com. White stained glass available at Stained Glass Supply, 2104 Colorado Blvd., Eagle Rock, CA 90041, 323-254-4361.

Lobster Thermidor: Rectangular (13" x 8") porcelain platter available exclusively at Sur La Table, 161 West Colorado Blvd., Pasadena, CA 91105, 626-844-2917. For the store nearest you, call 800-243-0852 or visit

www.surlatable.com. Small (6" x 6") porcelain plate and stainless steel "Oona" spoon by Cambridge (5-piece place setting only) available at Crate & Barrel, 75 West Colorado Blvd., Pasadena, CA 91105, 626-683-8000. For the store nearest you, call 800-323-5461 or visit www.crateandbarrel.com. Antique damask linen tablecloth (asst.) available at Bountiful Harvest, 1335 Abbot Kinney Blvd., Venice, CA 90291, 310-450-3620.

Miso Chicken Skewers: Imported "White Ruffle" oval platter available at Crate & Barrel, 75 West Colorado Blvd., Pasadena, CA 91105, 626-683-8000. For the store nearest you, call 800-323-5461 or visit www.crate andbarrel.com. Antique crocheted and cotton tablecloth (asst.) available at Bountiful Harvest, 1335 Abbot Kinney Blvd., Venice, CA 90291, 310-450-3620.

Somer Frittata: Porcelain "Fusion White Fish" platter by Bernardaud available at Geary's of Beverly Hills, 351 North Beverly Drive, Beverly Hills, CA 90210, 310-273-4741 or 800-793-6670, www.gearys.com. Antique embroidered and voile tablecloth (asst.) available at Bountiful Harvest, 1335 Abbot Kinney Blvd., Venice, CA 90291, 310-450-3620. Flowering herbs by Country Fresh Herbs, 18211 Emelita Street, Tarzana, CA 91356, 818-345-8810.

Roasted Mushrooms with Spinach, Cheese, and Pancetta: Imported French porcelain "Fusion Two-Section" server available at Williams-Sonoma, 142 South Lake Blvd., Pasadena, CA 91101, 626-795-5045. For the store nearest you, call 800-541-1262 or visit www.williams-sonoma.com. Antique crocheted and cotton tablecloth (asst.) available at Bountiful Harvest, 1335 Abbot Kinney Blvd., Venice, CA 90291, 310-450-3620.

Rock Shrimp Salad on Cucumber Rounds: BIA/ Cordon Bleu porcelain "Yin-Yang" dish (two pieces) available at Surfas, 310-559-4770, www.surfas

online.com. Antique linen and lace (asst.) available at Bountiful Harvest, 1335 Abbot Kinney Blvd., Venice, CA 90291, 310-450-3620.

Seared Tuna with Cilantro-Orange Sauce: Ramekin and "Butterfly" porcelain plate by Nambe available at De Vine Corporation, 732-751-0500, www.devine corp.net. Antique linen tablecloth available at Bountiful Harvest, 1335 Abbot Kinney Blvd., Venice, CA 90291, 310-450-3620.

Summer Salad on a Skewer: Small rectangular frosted-glass serving dish available at Maison Midi, 148 South La Brea, Los Angeles, CA 90036, 323-935-3157. French silver skewer "Martini Picks" (set of six) by Ercuis Silver imported by De Vine Corporation, 732-751-0500, www.devinecorp.net. Antique damask tablecloth (asst.) available at Bountiful Harvest, 1335 Abbot Kinney Blvd., Venice, CA 90291, 310-450-3620.

Melted Burrata Cheese with Roast Eggplant and Basil in Parmesan Cups: Imported "Varanges Camil" plate available at Maison Midi, 148 South La Brea, Los Angeles, CA 90036, 323-935-3157. Antique crocheted tablecloth (asst.) available at Bountiful Harvest, 1335 Abbot Kinney Blvd., Venice, CA 90291, 310-450-3620. Herbs by Country Fresh Herbs, 18211 Emelita Street, Tarzana, CA 91356, 818-345-8810.

Artichoke Leaves with Tarragon Aïoli and Shaved Parmesan: BIA/Cordon Bleu square "Sushi" plate available at Surfas, 310-559-4770 or www.surfasonline.com.

Antique pull-stitch linen and crochet with reindeer edge (asst.) tablecloth available at Bountiful Harvest, 1335 Abbot Kinney Blvd., Venice, CA 90291, 310-450-3620.

Seared Beef with Lime-Chili-Mint Dipping Sauce: BIA/Cordon Bleu porcelain "Sushiscape" sushi plate by Bret Bortner available at Surfas, 310-559-4770, www.surfasonline.com. Antique crocheted squares and cotton tablecloth (asst.) available at Bountiful Harvest, 1335 Abbot Kinney Blvd., Venice, CA 90291, 310-450-3620.

Sweet Shrimp with Hot Green Chutney: Ceramic earthenware "Petal" platter and appetizer plates and 3 oz. ramekin with grip (exclusively) available at Crate & Barrel, 75 West Colorado Blvd., Pasadena, CA 91105, 626-683-8000. For the store nearest you, call 800-323-5461 or visit www.crateandbarrel.com. Antique hand-crocheted and voile tablecloth (asst.) available at Bountiful Harvest, 1335 Abbot Kinney Blvd., Venice, CA 90291, 310-450-3620.

On the front cover: Imported "Scottish" martini glass by Christofle available at Christofle, 9515 Brighton Way, Beverly Hills, CA 90210, 310-858-8058, www.christofle.com. Silver martini picks by Ercuis Silver imported by De Vine Corporation, 732-751-0500, www.devinecorp.net. Small rectangular frosted-glass serving dish imported by Maison Midi, 148 South La Brea, Los Angeles, CA 90036, 323-935-3157.

Index

About the Author

SUZANNE SOMERS is the author of sixteen books, including the *New York Times* bestsellers *Keeping Secrets; Eat Great, Lose Weight; Get Skinny on Fabulous Food; Eat, Cheat, and Melt the Fat Away; Suzanne Somers' Fast and Easy; The Sexy Years;* and *Slim and Sexy Forever.* The star of the hit television programs *Three's Company* and *Step by Step,* Suzanne is one of the most respected and trusted brand names in the world, representing cosmetics and skincare products, apparel, jewelry, a computerized facial fitness system, fitness products, and a weight-loss program with a line of foods and appliances called Somersize. She received an honorary doctorate of humane letters from National University in California and is a highly sought-after commencement speaker.